M000233374

Ayurveda
for Life

Ayurveda for Life

Nutrition, Sexual Energy & Healing

Dr. Vinod Verma

SAMUEL WEISER, INC.

York Beach, Maine

First published in 1997 by
Samuel Weiser, Inc.
Box 612
York Beach, ME 03910-0612

Copyright © 1997 Vinod Verma
All rights reserved. No part of this publication may be reproduced or transmitted
in any form or by any means, electronic or mechanical, including photocopying,
recording, or by any information storage and retrieval system, without permission
in writing from Samuel Weiser, Inc. Reviewers may quote brief passages.

Library of Congress Cataloging-in-Publication Data
Verma, Vinod.
    Ayurveda for life : nutrition, sexual energy & healing / Vinod
Verma.
        p.   cm.
    Includes bibliographical references and index.
    ISBN 1-57863-009-6   (paper : alk. paper)
        1. Medicine, Ayurvedic.   2. Nutrition.   3. Sex instruction.
    I. Title.
R606.V47   1997
615.5'3—dc21   97-4947
                                                                         CIP

EB

Typeset in 11 point Baskerville

Cover: Amorous Krishna and Radha, while two musicians play music.
Rajasthani.

Printed in the United States of America

02   01   00   99   98   97
10 9 8 7 6 5 4 3 2 1

The paper used in this publication meets the minimum requirements
of the American National Standard for Permanence of Paper for
Printed Library Materials Z39.48–1984.

To all the Indian women
who have kept the Āyurvedic tradition alive
for thousands of years

NOTE TO READERS

The information provided in this book is not intended to replace the service of a physician. The material is presented for educational purposes and for self-help. The author and the publishers are in no way responsible for any medical claims regarding the material presented.

To use herbal or other remedial formulas described in this book for commercial purposes requires permission from the author. Write to the author in care of the publisher for more information.

TABLE OF CONTENTS

LIST OF ILLUSTRATIONS

PREFACE

Āyurveda is now familiar to many people in West. In bringing the practical wisdom of Āyurveda to the West, and in the process of teaching in Europe over the years, I have learned the difficulties, confusion, and misconceptions that Western students experience because of the rapid spread of Āyurveda. Some Westerners still look at the Āyurvedic wisdom from the point of view of modern medicine; that is, with a non-holistic and fragmented approach. Part of the problem has been caused by the fact that Āyurvedic wisdom is being taught by non-professional people, and many a time in an inappropriate manner. Ordinary people who genuinely want to follow the path of Āyurveda for longevity and health are sometimes misled. Āyurveda (the science of life) does not deal with the human body exclusively at a physical level, but includes the mental and spiritual levels simultaneously. The Āyurvedic way of life plays a foremost role in maintaining health and curing ailments.

Ancient Āyurvedic literature incorporates an extensive study on nutritional balance that is not only dependent upon the basic value of the nutrients, but is also related to time, place, and the fundamental nature (or *prakṛti*) of an individual. *Prakṛti* denotes both the physiological and mental characteristics of a person. The aim of Āyurveda is to attain a high quality life, optimum energy, longevity, and management of the numerous ailments and diseases human beings face. For the comprehension and application of various aspects of this ancient wisdom, one needs philosophical, as well as scientific and medical understanding.

Āyurveda cannot be equated with simplistic herbal therapy, where one learns which herb is good for which ailment. In Āyurveda, medicine and nutrition changed with time and space, and its fundamental scientific theories have stood the test of several thousand years. If we misinterpret or misrepresent this ancient theory, it can do us more harm than good. Following are a few examples of this in the context of nutrition. Several Āyurvedic books divide nutrients into three categories of the three humors (*vāta*, *pitta,* and *kapha*) and tell you to eat or avoid nutrients according to your body humors. For example, if you are a *kapha* type, or are dominant in this humor, you should avoid all foods which are *kapha*-promoting. A student in Munich once told me of a bad experience she had from misunderstanding this information. Realizing that she was dominant in *kapha,* she started avoiding all dominant *kapha* foods in her diet. She ended up in an extremely imbalanced situation, and became very nervous. She started having sleep disturbances.

We must understand that the body humors are not like glasses full or half full of a liquid, and that we can create balance by pouring something in or out. They are dynamic forces of the body; they are our energy and vitality, and we need them constantly. We cannot mathematically avoid nutrients pertaining to one humor to "create an equilibrium." Āyurvedic nutrition is more profound than this, and we students of Āyurveda should be aware that such a simplistic and naive approach will lead to ill health. We should be very critical and selective in choosing sources of information, as well as in choosing a teacher.

Another story which several students brought to my attention, both in Germany and Switzerland, was that someone lecturing on Āyurveda in these countries was emphasizing that Āyurveda advises to boil drinking water for at least an hour because by doing so it "changes its molecular structure and becomes very healthy." This statement is ridiculous from any scientific standard, for who can change the molecular structure of water? Water boiled for that length of time will have a high concentration of minerals in it, and, in the areas where water is hard, it will be damaging to the health, in addition to tasting awful.

Āyurvedic cooking is one of the two popular themes of Āyurveda, the other being *Panchakarma.* There are many Āyurvedic cookbooks available, but unfortunately they often deal simply with Indian cooking. You must keep in mind that all Indian cooking is not Āyurvedic, and many recipes given in these books are what Āyurveda will describe as anti-health. Some examples of forbidden things, or combinations that are erroneously described as Āyurvedic are: adding yogurt to meat preparations, or adding honey to hot drinks, or eating yogurt at night, or eating deep fried food too frequently or without appropriate precautions, such as adding particular spices to the food.

In my seminars and Āyurvedic cooking classes, I am often questioned about how to manage the cooking in a family if different members have different needs according to Āyurvedic instructions. The first and foremost approach to Āyurvedic cooking involves balanced meals which include a large variety of vegetables, fruits, and grains in order to have all the *rasas* in these foods (literally meaning taste, *rasas* are the basis of Āyurvedic pharmacology). Various Āyurvedic spices should be used to enforce equilibrium and create food that rejuvenates. As for the curative effect of food, different ailments, life conditions, and ages may need different compositions. There is a simple way of doing that in a family: after having cooked a balanced and rejuvenating food, you can add particular spices to it based on individual need, or for various curative effects. Spices are first put briefly in a spoonful of very hot ghee and cooked for a few seconds. For example, if you are an elderly person and complain of aches and pains, you need to add fenugreek, garlic, ginger, or heeng (asafoetida) in this manner into your soup, main dish, or whatever. If you feel the predominance of *kapha*, or the symptoms of it causing ill effects (lethargy, sleeping too much, a sweet taste in the mouth, etc.), you may add spices such as pepper, ginger, or garlic, while avoiding excessively fatty or sweet foods. If you have an excess of heat in the body, and tend to suffer from *pitta* disorders, add spices like anise, coriander, cardamom, and clove to your food.

In brief, I would like you to learn about Āyurvedic nutrition and cooking with wisdom, by observing the effect of various ingredients on your fundamental nature. You should slowly try to assimilate this mode of eating into your life. In this book, I provide the Āyurvedic values of individual food products, as well as some recipes. These will only initiate you into Āyurvedic cooking, and does not mean you should limit yourself to those recipes only. You should try to incorporate Āyurvedic wisdom in the food you habitually make by adding various spices and ingredients. I have also given the medicinal value of certain food products so that you can learn nutritional healing. For example, I have described that white gourd seeds strengthen the nerves and promote memory. You may add them to salads, or find other ways to incorporate them, in small amounts, in your food. You can write to me at the address given below in case you need more information about the availability of the products described here.

The second and third parts of the book discuss Āyurvedic concepts of sexuality and spiritual healing. However, while not well known in the West, this aspect of Āyurvedic wisdom is completely integrated in the Indian way of life. An integral view of holistic sexuality, simple remedies for sexual problems, and using aphrodisiacs or rejuvenating products will hopefully benefit modern men and women. Recognition of the infinite sexual energy present within all of us, and its beneficial channeling for healing and for a spiritual experience, are described in the last part of the book.

Āyurvedic healing and spiritual aspects are often ignored in many books on Āyurveda. According to Āyurvedic wisdom, just as we need to take constant care of the body to maintain our state of health, similarly the mind requires care. Negative qualities, like anger, greed, excessive attachment, and desire lead to many physical and mental ailments. We can maintain mental balance through breathing practices and concentration exercises popularly known as meditation. There are three humors, or vital forces (*vāta, pitta* and *kapha*) at the physiological level, and their equilibrium is essential for good health. Similarly the equilibrium of the three states of mind (*sattva, rajas* and *tamas*) is necessary for our well being and for evoking the subtle energy that lies dormant within us. *Tamas* are those qualities of the mind which hinder development. *Rajas* are the qualities relating to our daily activities, and *sattva* is the stillness of the mind. In our modern way of life, there is too much action and competition. Life is dominated by *rajas* and *tamas* qualities. *Sattva* is required to create a balance between *tamas* and *rajas*. It is *sattva* which leads us to discover the spiritual energy within all of us. I have described various simple mantras for evoking the spiritual energy, so we can use it beneficially for diagnostic and healing purposes.

This information has helped many of my European students to adopt an Āyurvedic way of life in the true sense. Comments and suggestions from readers are always welcome and will help me to further facilitate what I call "Āyurvedic communication."

Vinod Verma
The New Way Health Organization (NOW)
A-130 Sector 26, Noida 201310, India

ACKNOWLEDGMENTS

I have tried to compile in this volume the most common wisdom which has come to us through the ages. The concepts presented here are not taught in universities or colleges, but are assimilated from one's mother or grandmother, or just observed in life around us as we bloom from childhood to youth. Unfortunately, in these modern times, relationships are different due to our hectic pace, and this has hindered the smooth flow of our timeless wisdom. The advent of television has altered the course of our lives, and we are losing touch with the simple things in life. With these changing times, perhaps it is better to rethink how we communicate in order to let everyday wisdom flow again through the minds of our children and the generations to come.

In addition to my mother and late grandmother, I am most grateful to the following friends for their assistance in either stimulating the mind or helping me with their time and resources: Rupert Sheldrake, Kapila Vatsyayan, Elmar Gruber, Andrea Wolff-Biermann, Nancy Meyerson-Hess, and Eckhard Biermann. Figure 13 was drawn by Abhinav and Gayatri Verma, aged 10 and 7. They also appear in several photos.

I express my gratitude to my Āyurveda Professor, Priya Vrat Sharma, for his guidance in writing the Āyurvedic properties of individual food products.

I am indebted to Professor Rekha Jhanji for letting me use her own miniature paintings, as well as paintings from her private collection, to illustrate Part II.

Photographs of sculpture are gratefully acknowledged to the Archeological Survey of India.

—Dr. V. Verma

INTRODUCTION

Āyurveda has been recently introduced to the West through the media and because of our new interest in alternative health care. Āyurveda is an ancient medical system from India. However, Āyurveda is more than just a medical system, as it does not only deal with medicines and the cure of ailments. Curing ailments is one aspect, but Āyurveda actually deals with all aspects of life, and can be literally translated as "the knowledge or science of life." The word *Āyurveda* is constituted of two words: *ayus* and *veda*. The word *veda* literally means knowledge.[1] The conjunction of body, sense organs, mind and soul is called *ayus* or "life." Āyurveda can be said to deal with polarities—the good-bad or happy-unhappy aspects of life.[2]

Āyurveda involves the totality of life: pain and pleasure both form important aspects of this knowledge. On the one hand, we learn methods of getting rid of pain and sorrow, and on the other hand, we learn various ways to enhance the pleasures of life. We learn about human conduct and behavior, and the pain and pleasure originating from our conduct. Various environmental, nutritional, and behavioral aspects are taken into consideration in relation to their effect on our quality of life and longevity. Preventive health care methods are an important part of Āyurveda.

While learning about Āyurvedic methods of health care, there are two important factors to understand. First, Āyurveda views life as a totality; physiological, psychological, environmental, and spiritual

---

[1] Vedas are the ancient books of wisdom of the Hindus. There are four principal vedas which are over 3500 years old. They are *Ṛg, Yajur, Sāma* and *Athārva*. Āyurveda was made later as a separate veda. The earlier accounts on medicine are found in *Ṛg* and *Athārva* vedas.

[2] *Caraka Saṃhitā, Sūtrasthāna*, I, 41. Caraka wrote his book circa the seventh century B.C. In ancient times, the sages never wrote their names on their books, but these texts were gathered together by students. This translation by Prof. Priya Vrat Sharma.

aspects are interconnected, interrelated, and interdependent. Human beings, in their entirety, represent the miniature form of the cosmos, and changes in our environment (weather, climate, eclipses, tides, pollution, etc.) affect human life and health. Similarly, our actions affect our environment and bring changes to it. Life is considered in all its dimensions, and nothing is ignored. Because everything is interconnected and interdependent, food, sex, conduct, relationships, social behavior, and environment are all just as important as instructions to get rid of digestive disorders, depression, madness, anger, and so on. Therefore, we can say that Āyurveda is holistic. However, I would like to explain why Āyurveda is holistic and what is meant when we use the word. In recent years, the term "holistic" has been very loosely used in the West. Under this name, many Oriental techniques and other exotic methods for health care have gained popularity. Herbal medicine, herbal hygiene products (such as toothpastes, shampoos, soaps, and cosmetics of natural origin) are advertised as being natural and "holistic." I am speaking more to the holistic attitude when I use the word.

In modern Western medicine, the human body is only considered in parts. A sickness is analyzed at the molecular and micro level, and the cure is offered by chemical intervention. In a holistic system of medicine, medicine is not separately viewed from the rest of the life. It is not possible to visualize holistic medicine without having a holistic attitude toward life. This will soon be clear when I explain a little more about Āyurveda. Life is viewed in terms of cosmic unity. However, in Āyurveda, it is considered that we human beings are a part of the "whole" which is this cosmos. The cosmos is an ever-changing dynamic whole where nothing is purposeless. Everything has a purpose and a goal. Nothing is wasted; all things are transformed from one state to another. Since everything is interrelated and interconnected, no aspect of human existence can be taken independently without its affecting the other factors and vice versa. Thus, from a holistic point of view, when we are talking about health, we can not separate it from its other innumerable contexts. (See figure 1 on page xix.)

On the following pages, I will give you a brief exposition of the fundamental basis of Āyurveda which will make the comprehension of the rest of the text easier and will make it easy to adopt Āyurvedic methods.

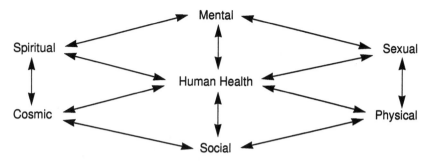

Figure 1. Human health in a holistic context.

In Āyurveda, the five fundamental elements (ether, air, fire, water, and earth) form the material reality of this universe. They are organized in a variety of forms, shapes, and proportions to form this beautiful world. What brings life to the material universe is the Universal Soul which pervades each element of the cosmos. The Universal Soul is without any substance; it is unchangeable; it is the animating principle of the Cosmic Substance. It is only energy. The real self of an individual is called *jīva*, or the soul, which is a part of the Cosmic energy or the Universal Soul. Unlike our material bodies, *jīva* is changeless and immortal. The body undergoes the transformation of birth, childhood, youth, old age, and death. After death, the five elements of the body go back to their main pool. That means they are organized in a certain fashion which renders us a particular form, and when the soul, or *jīva*, leaves this physical body, this latter disintegrates, and its five constituting elements separate. The *jīva* acquires another body and is said to be reborn. Thus, an individual soul undergoes a cycle of life and death. The past *karma* (the deeds of the previous life) are said to account for the quality of the next life.

Although we are born with certain given conditions and bodily constitutions due to our past karma, with our present karma, we can lessen the effect of our past karma. The essence of Āyurvedic practice lies in making every effort to maintain good health or to improve from weak or ill health. The following description will help you to understand the basic principles.

All physical functions of the body are governed by the three humors: *vāta*, *pitta*, and *kapha*. (You must remember the names because it is not possible to translate them.) I have mentioned that the whole of the universe is constituted of the five fundamental elements. This is at the material level. When the *jīva* enters the body made of five elements, the body starts living, and the five elements acquire the form of three vital forces in the body for the performance of all the body's physical and mental functions (*vāta, pitta, kapha*). Now let us see how the three humors are related to the five elements. Ether and air make *vāta*. *Pitta* is derived from fire. Water and earth constitute *kapha*. (See figure 2 below.)

The characteristics of these humors are similar to the elements from which they are derived. You can observe these elements in the cosmos. In your body, these elements represent cosmic reality. The vastness of the cosmos is limited within space and time in the human body. Let us see how this is done in the functional sense.

Ether and air are all-pervasive, light, dry, mobile, subtle, cold, and rough. *Vata* has similar characteristics. The functions of the body that involve movement and which are all-pervasive, are performed by *vāta*. Body movements, blood circulation, respiration, excretion, speech, sensation, touch, hearing, feelings like fear, anxiety, grief, enthusiasm, etc., natural urges, formation of the fetus, sexual urges, and retention are all *vāta* functions.

Pitta is hot, sharp, sour, and pungent. It is similar to fire. It is responsible for digestion, hunger, thirst, vision, heat regulation, softness, luster, cheerfulness, intellect, and sexual vigor.

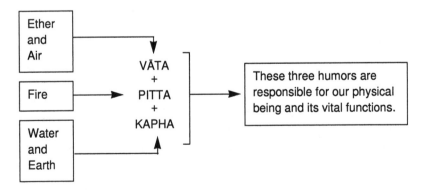

Figure 2. The three humors and their relationship to the five basic elements.

Water and earth give rise to *kapha,* which is cold, immobile, heavy, sweet, dull, and solid. *Kapha* constitutes the solid structure of the body, firmness and heaviness, sexual potency, forbearance, and restraint.

When in a state of balance and harmony, the five elements of the cosmos are life-supporting, whereas their imbalance causes destruction and catastrophe. Similarly, for a state of well-being, it is essential to maintain the equilibrium of these three humors. Just as the life-giving air, in the form of fast wind and tempest, can uproot trees and destroy houses, an excess of *vāta* gives rise to a number of specific disorders in the body. In normal conditions, the Sun helps plants grow, but a long and excessively hot summer brings drought, burns crops, and causes destruction. Fire gives us warmth, cooks our meals, but in a state of imbalance, fire can destroy life and property within minutes. Balanced *pitta* in the body gives timely hunger and thirst, appropriate body heat, etc., whereas, excessive *pitta* becomes the cause of another set of ailments in the body. The life-giving water of a river destroys crops, houses, and lives when there is a flood. An earthquake can be terribly devastating. Similarly, excessive *kapha* in the body leads to a third category of disorders.

The cosmos is a dynamic whole which is constantly changing. Nothing is static. There is night after day and day after night. Seasons follow each other, and each season brings us a variety of different fruits and vegetables. Similarly, our nature, behavior, and habits differ according to seasons and age. Even during one season, we face variations in weather that affect our physiological functions (like blood pressure, digestion, etc.) and our emotional state (cheerfulness, depression, anger, etc.).

An individual is born with a certain constitution which is determined by the domination of one humor or the other. I will try to explain, in a very simple manner, what the basic constitution is. All of us observe the differences in the basic behavioral patterns and the physiological reactions of people. Some of us work faster than the others, some feel better in summer, and others feel better in winter. For others, Spring may be the worst time of the year, because it brings discomfort from various ailments. According to Āyurveda, all of us relate differently to weather conditions, nutrients, life circumstances like grief, happiness, stress, etc., due to variations in our fundamental nature or *prakṛti.* For the details of humors and the basic constitution, the reader may consult my book on Āyurveda.[3] For maintaining good health, an equilibrium must be maintained. Everything we eat, drink, experience; our age, the climate, the weather, our life style, the type of work we do, and all other aspects of our existence constantly alter our humoral composition. The fundamental aim of Āyurveda is to teach us various ways to keep the balance. The balance saves us from inborn disorders, as well as making us strong enough to face external attacks. The equilibrium of the humors is also connected with mental balance and both are essential for complete harmony.

The mind has three different qualities (*rajas, tamas,* and *sattva*), and their balance is also essential for the balance of humors. In other words, there is an interrelationship between the six dimensions of one's being at both physical and mental levels. Thinking, working, making decisions, and everything associated with action and movement belong to the *rajas* quality of the mind. For example, a work day is predominatingly *rajas.* All that hinders action, ends motion, and hinders mental progress are of the *tamas* quality of the mind. Sleeping, sitting aimlessly without doing anything, or harboring feelings like jealousy, greed, etc., are *tamas* activities of the mind. Doing good deeds selflessly and without expectation, bringing the mind to stillness with yogic and meditative practices, and other deeds in this direction, belong to *sattva* activities.

Excessive *rajas* leads to *vāta* imbalance. Sleep is predominantly *tamas,* but people who lead hectic lives, talk too much and too loud, or watch too much television, have sleep that is restless and their minds do not rest, even during sleep. Thus, the equilibrium in activity and non-activity is not maintained. On the contrary, people who have nothing much to do, who sleep or daydream excessively, or who waste energy in harboring negative feelings are predominant in *tamas,* leading to an imbalance of *kapha.* The third dimension of the mind, *sattva,* is very important, and it should be integrated in *rajas* and *tamas* to bring a balance of mental activities for one's well-being. These three activities and their equilibrium are discussed in Part III of this book.

---

[3] V. Verma, *Ayurveda: A Way of Life* (York Beach, ME: Samuel Weiser, 1995).

Based upon the fundamental principles of Āyurveda, the present book deals with three important aspects that form an essential part of our day-to-day existence. In fact, these three parts are three different steps that take us from "external" to "internal." We begin with the "substance" and slowly move to the realm of energy beyond material reality.

Nutrition plays a very important role in keeping balance. An appropriate Āyurvedic diet depends upon the intrinsic quality of the food we consume, and should be coordinated to the basic constitution, age, season, time of the day, state of health, and geographical location. Food should be taken in the appropriate quantities. All these factors are interrelated and interdependent.

Āyurveda deals extensively in preventive methods for keeping good health. Food is important, and nutrients are evaluated according to humoral qualities. A nutrient may increase or decrease a particular humor, and the same nutrient may alter its humoral character according to its mode of preparation. In this respect, you will realize that Āyurveda has an entirely different view on nutrition than what you are used to. We don't deal with caloric values, minerals, proteins, carbohydrates, lipids, vitamins, etc. Āyurveda does not describe the qualities of foods as good, extremely good, or bad. All products can be harmful or useful, depending upon their preparation, time of consumption, and other factors. Food products are described as wholesome or unwholesome, and the latter require special attention to their preparation to get rid of unwholesome effects.

The importance of wholesome nutrition should also be understood in terms of enhancing the *ojas* (immunity and vitality) of the body. According to Āyurveda, the essence of absorbable food is distributed to the various organs *(dhatus)* of the body, which in turn make *ojas* with their activity. An effort should be made to enhance *ojas* because it helps prevent ailments, enhances one's physical and mental capability, and has a rejuvenating effect. The food comes from the five elements, in the form of the six *rasas* (literally meaning taste). Each *rasa* consists of two elements. The wholesome food should be enriched with all the *rasas* to provide the body with all five elements it needs. These in turn gives rise to the three vital forces (*vāta*, *pitta*, and *kapha*). The purpose of all this explanation is to illustrate that the balance of the humors is only one aspect for a healthy and fulfilled life.

Health in Āyurveda does not mean just a smooth functioning body. It is the total fulfillment of personality and harmony with the environment. Imagine a man who looks perfectly healthy to you. He has no health complaints in the usual sense of the word. He eats well, sleeps reasonably well, and evacuates properly. All his friends and acquaintances may think he enjoys good health. However, this person may be having some little problems that he doesn't talk about. He eats regularly and digests well, but he doesn't have a real appetite. Similarly, another person who looks equally healthy may have some subtle sexual problems. The problems of the first one may be cured by altering the order of his food and by adding *pitta*-enhancing substances to his diet. The problems of the second may also originate from diet, or from a lack of smooth distribution of the energy in his body due to a vitiated *vāta*. Āyurveda will not consider these people completely healthy. It offers a variety of comprehensive methods to enhance the capacity of the body for the fulfillment of all aspects of life. Since it is a unique feature of Āyurveda to deal extensively with human sexuality, I have chosen to discuss this in Part II of this book. The special aspects dealt with in Part II are nutrition, the performance of rituals to stop mechanization, and making sexual experience a conscious experience.

The dichotomy between the body and the mind is strongly prevalent in our modern times. The system of modern healthcare and present-day science and technology is based upon an ideology that originated in Western Europe only three hundred years ago. Philosophers and scientists asserted that this universe is like a mechanical system and so is the human body. Just as a machine made of various parts can be repaired by changing parts, similarly, our physical ailments can be treated. The ancient holistic view of life, nature, and the cosmos was slowly replaced by a mechanistic view of life.[4]

Do you feel like a machine? Indeed, many of us live like machines. We look at a day, not from the changing positions of the sun and its diminishing light in the evening, the onset of stars, and fall of the night, but with the movements of two hands on a clock, or the numbers on a watch. We have forgotten to feel the

---

[4] Rupert Sheldrake, *The Rebirth of Nature: The Greening of Science and God* (London: Century, 1990).

day. The same is true with the changing seasons. I was especially struck with this mechanical living during my stay in the United States when I was a research scientist at the National Institutes of Health (NIH) in Bethesda. The research building where I was working was constructed in such a way that no daylight entered the work area. This was an unacceptable situation for me and for three years, I could not get used to it. However, people around me could not understand my desire and inner need to look at time passing on something other than a watch. I was told that during work, one does not need to look outside. The second striking experience was about the seasons. Autumn on the East coast of the U.S. is very beautiful. In the large complexes of NIH, which spread over hundreds of acres, there were beautiful old trees and a very nice landscape frequented by birds. It was striking that the people passing by were so indifferent to this beauty. It seemed that nobody had the time to look up and admire the beautiful leaves turning red, or watch the exquisite birds chirping on their branches. To my utter surprise, in the city, there were organizations that offered Sunday tours for bird-watching or autumn leaves-watching. I want to say that with our dichotomized existence, we are growing increasingly distant from ourselves and from our surroundings.

Healing, which forms Part III of this book, is based upon the principle of bringing the mind back to this beautiful creation of nature—the human body—and concentrating it there. Some people in the West think that healing is something fantastic and mysterious. It might seem so to those who lead their lives at the direction of a clock or calendar, and who are unable to know themselves or to develop a communication with the physiological and mental functions. We need to develop awareness of our being, and an ability to withdraw our mind from the world, in order to concentrate the thoughts and the inner energy (*jīva*) on various physical and mental activities. We need to learn this, and we all have the capability and capacity to do that. We do not need special powers for healing ourselves or healing others. The special power is *jīva*, which is the same within each human being. To learn how to heal we need a strong desire to learn and persistence in our aim.

I have chosen these three subjects for this book because they concern our day-to-day existence. Āyurvedic knowledge can provide us with simple guidelines to improve our life style. However, this book does not make a complete guide to an Āyurvedic way of living. Neither does it provide you with the historical and technical background of Āyurveda. For all these aspects, readers may consult my other book on Āyurveda, which also provides details of the individual constitution, hygiene, treatment of minor disorders, and other features which concern our daily life.

PRONUNCIATION OF SANSKRIT

There are different ways to pronounce Sanskrit words, and here we will list the alphabet, the vowels, and the consonants. The accents that have been carried in this text indicate the special ways that this phonetic language is pronounced.

The Alphabet

a ā, i ī, u ū, ṛ, ṝ, ḷ, e ai, o au

k kh g gh ṅ

c ch j jh ñ

ṭ ṭh ḍ ḍh ṇ

p ph b bh m

y r l v

ś ṣ s

h

ṃ

ḥ

Vowels

a—a in America or o in come

ā—a in far or in father

i—i in pit or in pin

ī—ee in feel or i in machine

u—u in put or pull

ū—u in rule

ṛ—properly *ur*, but by modern Hindus as *ri* in river or in writ. *Ṛta (Rita), Ṛg Veda (Rig Veda), Prakṛti (Prakriti), Kṛṣṇa (Krishna)*.

e—ay in say or a in made

ai–i in rite or ai in aisle

o—o in go

au—ou in loud

Consonants

Consonants are pronounced approximately as in English, except for the following:

g—g in gun or in get (always "hard")

c—ch in church

sh (ṣ, ś)–sh in sheet or in shun

When *h* is combined with another consonant (e.g., th, bh), it is aspirated: *th* as in boathouse; *ph* as in uphill, etc. The palatal *ñ* is like the Spanish señor (*jña*, however, is pronounced most often by modern Hindus as "gyah," with a hard g).

PART I

AYURVEDIC NUTRITION

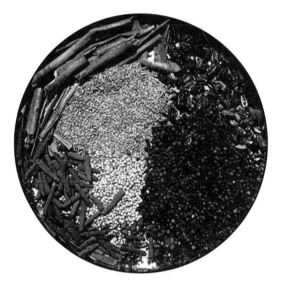

Āyurvedic spices.

Food provides vitality to all living beings; that is why people rush to food. Life, complexion, cheerfulness, good voice, imagination, happiness, contentment, corpulence, strength, intellect; all these are dependent on food. Worldly activities are done for livelihood, . . . and spiritual activities for the final liberation also depend on food.

Caraka Saṃhitā, Sūtrasthāna, XXI, 349–350
Sixth century B.C.

1

ĀYURVEDIC
NUTRITIONAL CONCEPTS

FOOD IS THE SECOND of the three principal vital factors for sustaining life; the first being breathing and the third, sleep. There is a tremendous variety of nutrients in the world, and during the last half century, biological and technological research has added further to the countless food items already existing. Bio-agriculture has offered us new varieties of grains, fruits, vegetables, etc. Some new hybrid varieties have invaded the market in the past decade. With increasing communication and travel, everything is grown everywhere, and when climate does not permit, food is grown under artificial climatic conditions. Many fresh vegetables and fruits are flown from developing countries to rich countries where people eat very varied diets.

In this century, we have successfully eradicated many epidemics with our latest developments in science and technology, through better hygienic methods, and through preventive health care—like vaccinations. However, diseases originating from food and environmental pollution have shown a sharp rise. Problems on our globe are made worse by a tremendous increase in population on the one hand, and an uneven distribution of wealth based on economic imbalances on the other. All this has resulted in an increase in diseases caused by malnutrition.

It is a general misconception in the affluent West that people are suffering from malnutrition only in the poor countries. Not getting all the essential nutrients for keeping healthy is only one part of malnutrition. Consuming more food than needed, not eating according to age, time, place, climate, and eating improper combinations form the other aspects of malnutrition, and it is this malnutrition that is prevalent in affluent societies. Besides, in the highly industrialized nations, eating has become a rapid, mechanical act, rather than a pleasurable, social, and conscious act. The American way of fast foods, and standing while eating, is rapidly catching up with the rest of the world.

The quality, quantity, method of preparation, way of consuming, the place, the time, etc., all play an important part in the effect that food has on us. Therefore, all these factors are of tremendous importance from an Āyurvedic point of view. The balance of nutrients in Āyurveda is considered in reference to the three humors. For strength, physical and mental equilibrium, and longevity, it is essential to maintain a balance between the three humors. What we eat and drink (including inhaling and smoking) constantly affects the body's humors. The way food is prepared, the way it is consumed, the timely or untimely intake, and how we combine different nutrients have a varied effect on us. For example, a rapidly gulped down meal, which is not properly chewed, will vitiate *vāta.*

Similarly, food preparation plays an important role. Cooking, in some cases, alters the humoral qualities as compared to raw food. Some foods may be good to eat in the morning, whereas their consumption at night may vitiate the humors. Each season has a particular dominating humor, and the choice of food should be varied in coordination with the seasons. Combinations of different foods may be harmful or beneficial. In some cases, certain nutrients which tend to increase or decrease a particular humor can be converted into a balanced food by the addition of certain spices. Last, food should be consumed according to our basic constitution. The basic constitution is determined by observing certain physiological and behavioral patterns.

To comprehend this holistic way of nourishment, and to be able to follow its principles in our day-to-day existence, requires a three-step program. The first step will be to gather information about harmonious nutrition in relation to time, place, quality, and quantity, the basic constitution, etc. The second step involves consciousness of these concepts, so we can relate them to our day to day existence. The third and the last step will deal with practical aspects and recipes. A wholesome diet requires that all three steps should be followed.

THE HUMAN
CONSTITUTION AND THE THREE HUMORS

Let me first explain the humoral concept of balance. It has been already said that according to Āyurveda, the three humors—*vāta, pitta,* and *kapha*—are responsible for all functions of the body. For maintaining good health, it is absolutely essential to keep balance between these humors. This balance is constantly altered by external factors, such as environment, nutrition, life style, etc. People who desire good health and long life will make every effort to maintain a harmony in the three humors. A humoral imbalance gives rise to many diseases which can be categorized with the humors. Diseases are caused due to vitiation of the humors. You may have more than one humor vitiated, and may suffer from inborn disorders from more than one category. An equilibrium of three humors not only saves you from inborn disorders, but also makes you resistant to external problems with viruses, bacteria, etc. In other words, the humoral equilibrium increases your immunity and gives rise to a strong constitution. Let us visualize the humoral concepts with figures.

Figure 1 (page 6) illustrates this balance. It is a triangle that represents the body and mind. The three arms of the triangle represent the three humors, and the circle in the center represents the soul, which is the cause of consciousness and the cause of our being. A healthy person with a strong constitution will have all the sides of the triangle equal (figure 1a); whereas a person with a weaker constitution will have three sides of the triangle in varying lengths. (See figure 1b–d). These are extreme examples. A large majority of people have one or two humors slightly dominating, or will have a sensitivity toward domination. This tendency of domination of a particular humor (or two humors) is responsible for the fundamental nature, or constitution (*prakṛti*) of a person. There are seven types of constitutions described in Āyurveda: *vāta, pitta, kapha, vāta-pitta, vāta-kapha, pitta-kapha* and *samdoṣa* (a balance of all three humors, as shown in figure 1a). The variation in the humors is responsible for the large variety of humoral nature among human beings.[1]

---

[1] See my other book, *Ayurveda: A Way of Life* (York Beach, ME: Samuel Weiser, 1995), Introduction, reference 4.

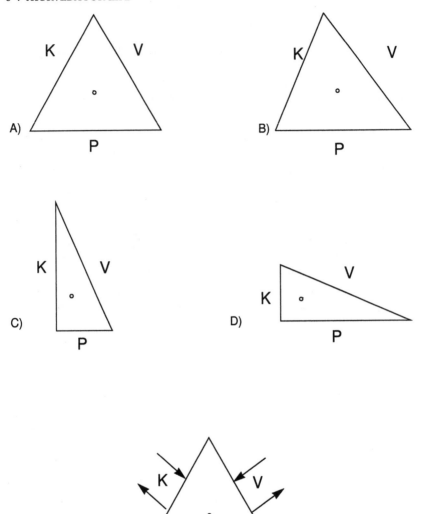

Figure 1. Balancing the humors: a) all the sides of the triangle are equal, representing that all the three humors are in equilibrium; b) vāta and pitta are slightly more than kapha, thus representing a state of a little imbalance; c) shows a state where pitta is very low (with the shorter arm of the triangle), thus representing a situation of extreme imbalance; d) kapha is very low when compared to vāta and pitta, thus representing another category of imbalance; e) shows that the humors are constantly influenced by external factors, and they alter with time, place, nutrition, our behavior, weather, climate, etc. Living in harmony with our surroundings will help us maintain a healthy balance.

The external factors keep altering the humors (see figure 1e on page 6). That is where our freedom lies. We can harmonize these factors to a large extent, and change ourselves from unhealthy to healthy, from weak to strong, or the contrary. This is the basis of our effort for good health and a long life. Right nutrition plays a major role in maintaining good health, making people with weak constitutions stronger and healthier, and curing minor disorders with nutritional therapy.

Let us first look at the principal features that help you determine your humoral nature, or basic constitution. This is the first step before proceeding to the effect of various foodstuffs on your humors. I will describe some principal characteristics of the various constitutions. You may feel that you fall very slightly in one category. However, at times these characteristics are enhanced. This indicates that your humors are in balance and you are a healthy person, but you have a bit of a tendency for dominance of that particular humor. With an imbalanced diet which promotes that particular humor, the mild symptoms become strong, and they might be disturbing, or become the cause of ailments. Some other individuals may have only some of the given characteristics of a particular humor. It is also possible that you may find you have the characteristics of two humors simultaneously. It means that you have a dominating tendency for two humors. Now, let us see what *vāta-*, *pitta-*, and *kapha*-dominating people are like.

If you tend to be rather agile, swift in action, quick in fear, or other emotions, if you get irritated easily, are not tolerant to cold, shiver easily, then you are certainly a *vāta*-dominated person. The *vāta*-dominated person may also have prominent blood vessels and coarse hair and nails.

As you know, *pitta* is derived from the basic element fire, and *pitta*-dominating people are intolerant of heat, perspire a lot and usually have a hot face. They have a lustrous complexion, excessive hunger and thirst, body odor, are generally intolerant, and lack endurance.

Quite opposite to the *vāta*-dominated person, the *kapha* person is slow and stable, and speaks less than others. This type is slow to react. In contrast to a *pitta*-dominated person, the *kapha* person is not hungry and thirsty, and perspires very little. The eyes are clear and so is the complexion.

By observing yourself carefully, you can determine if you have one or two dominating humors, or if you are a person with harmonious humors. Once you are able to determine your basic constitution, it will be easy to work on yourself. Finding your constitution is the starting point for learning a nutritional balance. The secret is to keep the dominating humor or humors in balance with diet. By doing the reverse out of ignorance, that means, by enhancing the dominating humor further through incorrect nutrition, you let this humor vitiate. The vitiation of a particular humor will cause related disorders.

NUTRITION IN RELATION TO TIME, SEASON, AGE, AND PLACE

In the holistic system of Āyurveda, you have to learn to relate your nutrition to your constitution as well as to the environment. First of all, let us explore the relationship of humors to time in terms of day, year, and life in order to relate them to the intake of food.

Figure 2 (page 9) shows various parts of the twenty-four hour day in relation to the humors. The time used in the figure is approximate, as in Āyurvedic literature, time is indicated by duration measured according to the position of the Sun. In this figure, I have given time based on a 12 hour day and 12 hour night. You may adjust this time to summer and winter and to your particular geographical location. In Āyurvedic literature, this time is described as follows: *vāta* increases during the evening and the last part of the night, *pitta* is high around noon and midnight, whereas *kapha* is enhanced during the morning and the first part of the night.

Now let us see the humors in relation to various seasons of the year. Since this book may be used in any part of the world, I will not go by the calendar months. I will rather describe the weather conditions. Rain brings coolness and humidity, and the rainy season is *vāta*-inducing. Warm and dry weather (summer and also autumn in some parts of the world) is *pitta*-inducing. Cold climates (winter and spring) tend to aggravate *kapha*. Because of the varied humoral effects of the different seasons, the changing seasons sometimes have an ill effect on our health. Too

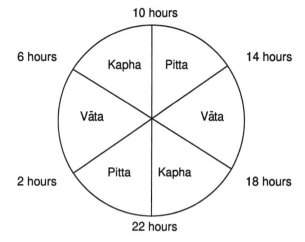

Figure 2. Various parts of the day in relation to humors.

much difference in day and night temperatures, or humidity, gives rise to humoral imbalance. This brings down the resistance and one tends to catch all sorts of infections and minor ailments during the time when seasons are changing.

During the lifetime, childhood is *kapha*-dominating, youth is *pitta*-dominating, whereas old age is marked by an increase of *vāta.*

Place also affects the humors. The forest is *vāta*-dominating, while deserts tend to enhance both *vāta* and *pitta.* Mountain regions are *vāta-* and *kapha*-dominating, whereas areas near the sea are *kapha-* and *pitta*-dominating. Midlands are said to have a very mild effect on humors.

The change of humors with respect to various external factors is shown in Table 1 on page 10.

VARIOUS CATEGORIES OF FOOD

According to Āyurveda, food can be divided into various categories in relation to its source, effect, way of intake, and taste. The following list makes this simple.

Table 1. The Humors and the Environment.

HUMORS IN RELATION TO SEASONS	
SEASON	DOMINATING HUMORS
Rainy	Vāta
Warm and Dry	Pitta
(Summer and Autumn)	
Cold (Winter)	Kapha
HUMORS IN RELATION TO AGE	
AGE	DOMINATING HUMORS
Childhood	Kapha
Youth	Pitta
Old Age	Vāta
HUMORS IN RELATION TO PLACE	
PLACE	DOMINATING HUMORS
Forest	Vāta
Desert	Vāta-Pitta
Mountains	Vāta-Kapha
Coastal Areas	Kapha-Pitta
Midlands	None

1. Food comes from the plant and animal kingdoms.

2. We can absorb food into our system by chewing it, drinking it, licking it.

3. Food has various properties. It can be viscous/liquid, heavy/light, cold/hot, unctuous/rough, dull/sharp, stable/mobile, soft/hard, slimy/non-slimy, smooth/coarse, minute/gross.

4. The food we use can be wholesome or unwholesome.

In Āyurvedic terms, wholesome food does not alter drastically the body humors. It is food that contains the three humors in equilibrium. The resultant material of the humors are the *dhātus* which circulate throughout the body, providing energy for all the physical and mental functions. Thus, a wholesome food is not harmful to the *dhātus* of the body. It does not block the energy channels. Unwholesome food has the contrary effect; it creates an imbalance, including the *dhātus*, and blocks the energy channels. Eating unwholesome food lowers the body's resistance by bringing down *ojas* and thus makes one vulnerable to disease.

Some foods that are naturally wholesome are a variety of rice called *śālī*, fresh green peas, carrots, natural rock salt (not the purified kind), ghee, cows milk, sesame oil, ginger, grapes, and products made from sugarcane. Other foods that are hard to digest are Urad dāl, potatoes, and mustard. This does not mean that one should not eat "unwholesome" foods. It means we should prepare them carefully by adding special spices and making combinations or preparations so the effect is no longer unwholesome. This subject will be discussed later.

2

FOOD IN
RELATION TO HUMORS

YOU HAVE LEARNED that everything affects our humoral balance. However, this effect cannot be measured in terms of absolute values as it depends upon the individual constitution, age, location, season, and nutrition. In Āyurveda, everything can be a medicine or a poison depending upon the circumstances. A few glasses of cold water, a dip in the pool, and some appropriate fruits can cure somebody's vitiated *pitta* and the same *pitta*, when it is not taken care of, can vitiate by inappropriate nutrition and lead to various ailments. Timely nutritional care can save us from hundreds of health problems, whereas the contrary can bring us to critical health conditions. Imagine someone who is *vāta*-dominated. He or she lives in the mountains and is quite careless about food. This person takes overripe, dry and *bāsā* (prepared well in advance) food, along with other *vāta*-promoting substances, like cauliflower and lentils, without making balanced preparations with the appropriate herbs and spices. This person will always suffer from aches and pains, body stiffness and/or restlessness, insomnia, etc. *Vata* plays havoc in his or her body, just as a stormy night uproots the trees and destroys property (remember that *vāta* is derived from the basic ether and air elements). Going further with this example, when this person enters the late 40s and early 50s, his or her problems enhance as this is the *vāta*-dominating age. All these factors combine and this person ends up with one or more *vāta* diseases, such as goiter, arthritis, nervous disorders, insomnia, high blood pressure, etc. Of course, there are factors other than nutrition which can worsen the vitiated *vāta*, like an exposure to cold, injury, excessive physical exercise, and so on. But in the present context, we are concerned with Āyurvedic nutrition.

I will now describe the humoral effect of some of the most common foods so you will be able to coordinate them with your basic constitution and environmental factors. I will provide a short description to help you to understand the fundamental principles of Āyurvedic nutrition. This is particularly essential today because there is a tremendous variety of food including basics like rice, yogurt, salt, milk, grains, etc. The description given will help readers make an appropriate choice.

I have divided the various foods into six major categories: 1) grains; 2) fruits and vegetables; 3) dairy products; 4) eggs; 5) herbs and spices; 6) miscellaneous.

GRAINS

Grains can be divided into two major categories. In the first category are the grains obtained from grassy plants like rice, wheat, barley, etc. These grains are used as staple foods in many parts of the world. The second category includes grains obtained from leguminous plants, like different varieties of beans. The common name in English is pulses, and in India, they are popularly known as "dāl."

Grains from Grassy Plants

Barley: Barley used to be the principal cereal of ancient India. Now it is used less. In the West, it is largely used to make beer. Barley flour can be used to make bread. Barley regulates *kapha*, but increases *vāta*.

Maize (corn in America): Maize originally comes from South America, but it is eaten all over the world. Maize grains are eaten in various forms, and maize flour is used to make bread, crêpes, tortillas, etc. Maize is dry by nature; it increases *vāta*, but decreases *kapha* and *pitta*.

Millet: There are many varieties of grains under this name. However, in Sanskrit and other Indian languages, they have different names. I will describe some important varieties. In India, these grains are used frequently, but in the West, you will generally find them only in health food stores.

Common millet (Sanskrit: *chīnāka*, Hindi, *chīnā* or *māḍhā*) increases *vāta* but regulates *kapha*.

Italian millet (*Kanguni* in Hindi) has the same Āyurvedic properties as the common millet.

Great millet (*Jūrṇa* in Sanskrit and *Javāra* in Hindi) can be eaten like rice after cooking in water. Its flour is used to make bread. It regulates *kapha* and *pitta*.

Finger millet (*Madhūlika* in Sanskrit and *Maḍuā* in Hindi) is a wholesome food, for it regulates all three humors and is good for curing vitiated *pitta*. In the Southern Indian state of Karnatka, finger millet is given to weak babies and to the mothers after childbirth for restoring health.

Rice: Rice is the world's most used food. There are several varieties of rice. Most rice is polished before selling. It is a general misconception in the West that all rice is brown before polishing and white after polishing. Many people think that the "brown rice" is more nourishing as the process of polishing removes certain nutrients. It is essential to learn that what is generally known as "brown rice" is a variety of rice which is brown! It takes a long time to cook; it is heavy to digest and increases *vāta*. Polished rice has lesser nutritional value but is easy to digest. Secondly, there is a variety of rice which is naturally white. The grains are small and rounded, and this variety of rice is known as *śālī* rice in Āyurvedic literature. It is considered to be the best. This rice promotes *vāta* and *kapha* very slightly, and decreases *pitta*. The other varieties of rice tend to promote *vāta* more. New rice is heavy to digest. One year old rice is best for consumption, whereas rice that is older than that is *vāta*-promoting. Wild rice is also *vāta*-enhancing.

Wheat: Wheat comes next to rice in its use in world nutrition. Like rice, wheat is used as staple food in many parts of the world and is also "cold" in its Āyurvedic nature. It decreases *pitta*. New wheat increases *kapha*, but old does not.

Grains from Leguminous Plants

Many of these grains are called by a common name in India—*dāl.* Dāls include different kinds of lentils and beans. Dāls are a popular source of proteins because many Indians are vegetarians. Besides, meat preparations are generally *pitta*-promoting, and because of the domineeringly hot climate, even non-vegetarians eat a limited quantity of meat. Therefore, a dāl preparation is generally used for one of the two meals. Āyurvedic texts suggest that dāls should not be taken for dinner as they are heavy to digest. It is also said that dāls should be prepared with spices and ghee in order to facilitate their digestion. A recipe for the preparation of dāl is described later. (See page 54.)

Chickpeas: Nearly every culture in the world uses the chickpea. There are two types—white and brown. The white variety is better known in the West. Both types of chickpeas bring down *pitta.* With ghee, they make a wholesome food and help balance vitiated humors. Germinated chickpeas (sprouts) are a wholesome food.

Chickpea flour is known as *basin,* and is available in Indian shops. You may also make it yourself from the grain. This flour is used for cleaning the skin, as has been described elsewhere.[1] Gram flour mixed with wheat flour makes a nourishing and wholesome food, and is used for making bread.

Green gram or mung beans (Hindi: *Moong Dāl***):** The Hindi name of these beans has become popular in the West and they are sold as moong beans (mung beans in the USA) in health food stores. They are also available in the Chinese shops.

According to Āyurvedic literature, this dāl is best of all the dāls as it is easy to digest and is a wholesome food. It brings all three humors in harmony. It is a protein, vitamin, and mineral-rich food, and is often given to sick and weak people.

This dāl is eaten in many forms—the entire grain, sprouts, slightly ground, with or without the skin. The skin is dull green, whereas the grains without skin are yellow. From the mung bean flour, many different sweet and salty dishes are made. However, this flour does not taste good when used for making bread.

---

[1] See my other book, *Ayurveda: A Way of Life* (York Beach, ME: Samuel Weiser, 1995), Introduction, reference 4.

Note: In recent years, scientists have developed many varieties of mung beans which are bigger in size and are *vāta*-promoting.

Green peas: Eaten all over the world, peas are sold fresh, frozen, as well as in dried form. Young peas are slightly *vāta*-promoting and they decrease *pitta*. But ripe and over-ripe peas increase *vāta* intensely. Like all other dāls, peas are protein rich and a nourishing food.

Masoor beans: These beans are known as lentils in many countries in the West. They are heavy to digest with the skins on, so it is recommended to use them partially crushed and without skin. Without skin, they are pink. In this form, they are available in health food stores, in Chinese shops, and sometimes in big city supermarkets.

This dāl increases *vāta*, whereas it decreases *pitta* and *kapha*. It is used with ghee to bring down vitiated *pitta*. A recipe for masoor dāl soup is included on page 55.

Soy beans: There are many varieties of soya beans all over the world and they are eaten in various forms. Soya beans are more rich in proteins than the other dāls. They are heavy to digest, strength giving, *vāta*-decreasing and *pitta*-promoting. They are easier to digest after germinating them slightly. Since soybeans are *pitta*-promoting, their flour mixed with wheat flour makes a wholesome diet.

Urad beans (Sanskrit, *Māsa*; Hindi, *Urad*): Urad dāl resembles green gram in size and shape, but it is black instead of green. As for the properties, they are quite different from the green grams, as this dāl is heavy to digest. It is an unwholesome food in that it increases both strong *pitta* and *kapha*. It brings down *vāta*. Because of its strong Āyurvedic qualities, special care should be taken for its preparation, otherwise it can make one sick. Its flour is easy to digest when mixed with rice flour, and this mixture is very commonly used in southern India for many food preparations.

Urad dāl has important medicinal qualities despite its unwholesome effect as a food. It cures impotency, increases sexual secretions and potency, helps enlarge breasts, and increases sexual desire. Some recipes are mentioned in the next section (see page 86). Because of these qualities, it is widely used in India in many forms.

Like the mung beans, Urad beans (black gram) is also used with or without the skin, and is partially crushed. In some recipes, especially in Part II, there is a mention of Urad dāl flour. This is generally not available ready made, but you can easily prepare it fresh in a small coffee grinder. You do not need large quantities of this flour in the recipes described here. Therefore, it is very convenient to make small quantities in a coffee grinder. It is recommended to keep one such grinder exclusively for Āyurvedic spices and other such preparations.

Outside the Indian continent, Urad beans are only available at Indian food stores. Perhaps because of its unwholesome effect, it is not available in the health food stores. Considering its medicinal qualities, our organization is making an effort to promote its availability and use.

• • •

There is a large variety of other dāls which I have not described for the sake of brevity. I have mentioned the most important and common ones. But before I close this subject, I want to name one dāl available in many countries which should not be eaten by animals or human beings. It is called grass peas or chickling peas (the Latin name is *Lathyrus sativus*, Sanskrit, *Triputaka*, and Hindi, *Khesari*). In Āyurvedic literature, it is described as extremely *vata*-promoting, constipating, and regular use leads to partial paralysis. We also know from modern research that it contains a poisonous chemical that slowly causes nerve damage.[2]

VEGETABLES, FRUITS, AND NUTS

Now I will describe some commonly eaten vegetables and fruits from all over the world. I will give instructions for possible combinations to help create a wholesome diet. The medicinal qualities of some vegetables and fruits are also discussed.

---

[2] Peter S. Spencer, et al. "Lathyrism: Evidence for Role of the Neuroexcitatory Aminoacid BOAA," *Lancet*, Nov. 8, 1986.

Vegetables

Aubergine (Eggplant): There are several different varieties of aubergine—small, round, elongated, etc. It is rich in vitamins and minerals, and increases *kapha* and *pitta*. Aubergine seeds promote *vāta* and that is why over-ripe aubergines cause an imbalance of all three humors. When the entire aubergine is roasted on a fire, or in the oven, before preparation, it becomes easy to digest, and does not cause an imbalance of the humors. Fried aubergines are not recommended.

Bitter gourd: It is called *Karela* in northern India. It is a spindle-shaped, green vegetable, measuring 4–5 inches in length. It has an uneven and engraved surface. As the name suggests, it is bitter to the taste. It is a summer vegetable in India, and is available in England, North America, and where Indian communities have settled. The reason I mention this vegetable is that it has many medicinal qualities. It is a preventive against diabetes, fevers, leucorrhoea, and *pitta* disorders. It purifies the blood and is beneficial for respiratory ailments. As a medicine, a teaspoon or two of the fresh juice is recommended. It may be eaten regularly as a vegetable. The bitter taste is overcome by cooking it with onions, ghee, and tomatoes. Bitter gourd (or *Karela*) is available only at the Indian shops in the USA. There is no other name for it in English. Its Latin name is *Momordia charantina*. It is probably grown in the southern USA to cater to the needs of the population from the Indian continent. It grows only in a very hot climate.

Brussels sprouts: This vegetable has properties like those of cabbage. In fact, they are a kind of cabbage which is smaller in size.

Cabbage: Widely used all over the world, cabbage is eaten raw as well as cooked. It is a strength-giving vegetable, but it is heavy to digest. It is "cold" in its Āyurvedic properties as it diminishes *pitta*. It also promotes *vāta*. Cook it with some tomatoes, lemon juice, or appropriate spices.

Carrots: These are wholesome vegetables and bring balance to the three humors in the body. Because of this quality, carrots are a good vegetable to mix with dāls and other vegetables. Carrots revitalize the heart and liver functions. They are also recommended to people suffering from piles, fevers, and stomach problems. Carrot seeds are used as contraceptives and for causing abortion.

Cauliflower: This vegetable is *pitta*-promoting and is heavy to digest. Thus, it is classified as a "hot" food in Āyurvedic terminology. It is said that cauliflower helps bring balance to an excess of *vāta* and *kapha*. However, experience shows that these properties are present in very small traditional varieties of cauliflower which are still grown by some farmers, but the hybrid varieties, which have the very big and "beautiful" flowers, are *vāta*-promoting. Therefore, it is advised to use a small amount of garlic and ginger in the preparation of cauliflower.

Cress (Watercress): Used mostly as salad, cress is slightly pungent in taste, and cures vitiated *vāta* and *kapha*.

Endive or Chicory: This is usually eaten as salad. It is a very good vegetable as it cures vitiated *pitta* and *kapha*. It is especially beneficial to cure a lack of appetite and to revitalize the liver functions.

Fennel: A European vegetable not used in India. It is especially good to cure a bad stomach and other digestive disorders. It has a healing effect on stomach ulcers. It is light to digest, promotes liver functions, and cures vitiated *pitta* and *vāta*.

Green beans (French beans): They increase *vāta* and decrease *kapha* and *pitta*. They should also be prepared with ginger or garlic or both. They also make a good combination with potatoes.

Okra: Also called lady's finger. It is rarely sold in continental Europe, but is a common vegetable in Asia and America, and is also sold in England. It is a very sticky vegetable, and should be washed and dried before cutting. Okra increases *kapha* but decreases *pitta* and *vāta*. It is heavy to digest and should not be taken excessively. It should be prepared with ginger.

Potatoes: Potatoes originate in South America, but they are a very popular food all over the world. They are strength-giving and are rich in minerals and vitamins. They should not be eaten indiscriminately, as they are heavy to digest, *vāta-* and *pitta*-promoting and may cause internal hemorrhaging. Potatoes also promote *kapha*; therefore, they should be selectively eaten with certain foods. It is not recommended to eat deep-fried potatoes. Since potatoes are a *pitta*-promoting food, it is best to cook them with ghee, which lessens their *pitta* effect. Potatoes should be boiled with the skin on. The skin may be removed before eating. After that, the potatoes may be roasted slightly with butter or ghee.

Radish: Small round radishes are more popular than the big white or black radishes. The small radish is a wholesome food and gives balance to the humors. Big radishes cure vitiated *vāta*. Over-ripe radishes, whether big or small, vitiate *vāta* and *pitta* and should be avoided. The big radish, along with its leaves, may also be cooked with spices. Radish juice is often given to people suffering from piles.

Spinach: This is another vegetable which is eaten nearly all over the world. It is very rich in iron and minerals. Contrary to potatoes, spinach is "cold" in its Āyurvedic properties, meaning that it diminishes *pitta*. It also brings down *kapha*. Its combination with potatoes makes a wholesome food. An excess of spinach causes distension, but this negative effect can be removed by cooking it with soybeans or chickpeas.

Tomatoes: Like potatoes, tomatoes are one of the most popular vegetables in the world, and are eaten raw in salads or cooked with other vegetables. Tomatoes are used to make sauces. Because of their sweet and sour character, tomatoes increase *kapha* and *pitta* slightly. Over-ripe tomatoes with big seeds are hard to digest. Otherwise, tomatoes are a light food and are strength-promoting. Freshly extracted tomato juice taken a little before meals cures lack of appetite.

Turnips: This vegetable is not eaten often in Europe. It is a wholesome vegetable, like the carrot, and causes humoral equilibrium. It is highly recommended to eat this vegetable.

White gourd melon: This is also known as pumpkin, but it is white inside, whereas pumpkins are yellow. It is eaten as a vegetable as well as a dessert in many different forms. It is a wholesome food if it is eaten when it is just ripe. It regulates the three humors. Young unripe pumpkins decrease *pitta*, whereas overripe ones increase it. Pumpkin is strength-giving, diuretic, laxative, and is especially good for revitalizing the functions of the heart and liver. The seeds cure vitiated *vāta* and *kapha* and strengthen the nerves. They are eaten as are other nuts—after removing the shells. They are recommended to people who have constant and chronic headaches. A daily dose of seeds should not exceed more than ⅛ ounce.

The yellow pumpkin is bigger in size than the white, and as the name suggests, it is yellow inside. It is heavier to digest compared to the white. It helps control vitiated *kapha* and *pitta*. It is also a laxative, like the white pumpkin.

Fruits and Nuts

Almonds: There are two types of almond—bitter and sweet. Bitter almonds are poisonous and contain hydrocyanides. They should not be eaten. Sweet almonds increase *kapha* and *pitta*, but they cure excessive *vāta*. Almonds should be avoided in hot climates and in *pitta* and *kapha* ailments. Almonds are an aphrodisiac and are strength-promoting.

Apples: Apples bring down *vāta* and *pitta*, but they increase *kapha*. Sour apples, however, increase *pitta*.

Apricots: Increase *kapha* and *pitta*, but regulate vitiated *vāta*.

Bananas: A heavy fruit to digest. They are "cold" in their Āyurvedic nature. Bananas increase *kapha*, but decrease *vāta* if the fruit is ripe. Slightly over-ripe fruits increase *vāta* and cause distension. Over-ripe bananas should be avoided.

Figs: Figs are "cold" in their Āyurvedic properties. They regulate excessive *vāta* and *pitta*.

Grapefruit: Because of its bitter qualities, in spite of being sour, grapefruit does not increase *pitta*. It helps cure vitiated *vāta*.

Grapes: Sweet and ripe grapes regulate vitiated *vāta* and *pitta*. They are beneficial in fever and weakness. Sour grapes, however, vitiate *pitta*. Dried grapes (raisins) are beneficial to cure coughs and bad throats. They are used in many Āyurvedic recipes along with other substances.

Guava: Guava regulates the vitiated *pitta* but increases *kapha* and *vāta*. It cleans the digestive tract and is diuretic.

Kiwi: The small black seeds of this fruit are highly *pitta*-promoting. Therefore, an excessive use of this fruit should be avoided.

Lemons: There are many varieties of lemon and the best is the sweet lime, which is smaller in size as compared to the citron generally sold in the West. Sweet lime is round and greenish yellow with a thin outer skin. In general, all lemons promote digestive power and cure vitiated *vāta* and *kapha*. Lemons are also good to cure excessive thirst, a dry mouth, and a dry throat. A regular use of lemon saves one from *vāta* and *kapha* ailments, and purifies the blood.

Litchis: Originally a Chinese fruit which is eaten all over Asia now. Because of the Chinese communities spread all over the world, this fruit has become popular almost everywhere. Litchis promote *pitta* and *kapha*, but it decreases *vāta*.

Mangoes: This fruit should be taken when appropriately ripened. Sour mangoes lead to vitiation of the humors, indigestion, boils, other skin problems, and eye ailments. A ripe, sweet fruit, however, is strength-giving, and regulates *vāta* and *pitta*. It also increases sexual potency.

Musk melon: Generally known as simply melon in the West, the musk melon is "cold" in its Āyurvedic qualities. It is a summer fruit. It brings down both *pitta* and *vāta*. It is diuretic, strength-giving, and increases sexual potency.

Oranges: Oranges and other similar fruits are rich in vitamins and minerals. They cure vitiated *vāta* and slightly enhance *pitta*. If the sour taste is dominating, they enhance *pitta*. If they are too sour, they should be eaten with salt or sugar.

Papaya: A very good fruit to cure vitiated *pitta*. It is specially recommended to cure stomach problems and for pregnant women.

Peaches and plums: These two fruits have similar Āyurvedic qualities. They are slightly *pitta*-promoting, but they regulate *vāta* and *kapha*.

Pears: "Cold" in Āyurvedic qualities. Pears have a mild effect on the humors, and are wholesome fruits.

Pineapple: Called *anānās* in Hindi and various other languages, this fruit is strength-giving, *vāta*-decreasing and *kapha*-promoting. It is a laxative, and freshly pressed pineapple juice has antibiotic and anti-parasitical qualities. It is specifically recommended for intestinal parasites.

Pistachios, Pine nuts, Cashews, and Walnuts: All these nuts have similar properties to almonds. *Caution:* All nuts should be avoided when suffering from colds, coughs, chest congestion, or asthma.

Pomegranates: The sweet-tasting, properly ripe fruits establish humoral equilibrium. However, the sour and unripe fruit promotes *pitta* and may also cause distension. Pomegranates are good for strengthening heart and brain functions.

Watermelon: This big green melon is red inside. It is heavy and "cold" in its Āyurvedic properties. Its excessive use is not good for the eyes. It is an anaphrodisiac. If over-ripe, it increases *pitta*.
Caution: Melon and milk are antagonists. Do not eat melon with milk. Combining milk and watermelon gives rise to distension, a bloated stomach, and other digestive problems.

DAIRY PRODUCTS

Butter and Ghee: Ghee is clarified butter (the preparation method is described on page 47). Both butter and ghee decrease *vāta* and *pitta*, and increase *kapha*. They promote strength, cure general weakness, increase intellect and potency. Ghee is used to cure an excess of *vāta* and *pitta*. It is also used in many Āyurvedic preparations as it enhances the effect of medicines. According to Āyurveda, ghee is the best of all cooking fats.

Cheese: In the West, there are many varieties of cheese, and it is an important part of the nutrition. Creamy, fresh varieties of cheese slightly promote *pitta* and *kapha*. The other more ripe varieties largely promote *pitta*. Cheese should be used in moderate quantity as it is a very rich food, and its excessive use leads to *pitta* vitiation and related disorders.

Milk: Āyurveda describes eight types of milk from different animals. But in the present description, we will limit ourselves to only cows' milk. Before describing the properties of the milk, it is necessary to add that pasteurized milk that can be preserved for several days certainly does not have those properties of fresh milk. The treated milk generally promotes *vāta*.

Cows' milk is considered the best and is a wholesome food. It cures vitiated *vāta* and *pitta*, increases the body's *ojas* (immunity), promotes strength, and is an aphrodisiac. Milk is "cold" in its Āyurvedic properties, and therefore the use of cold milk in summer and hot milk in winter is recommended. Hot milk has antifatigue qualities. Cows' milk is recommended to growing children and weak persons. Hot and sweetened milk promotes sleep.

Human milk is a wholesome diet which brings equilibrium to the humors. However, if the mother is careless and eats unwholesome foods, the properties of the milk change. Mothers should be careful during the lactating period, for when they eat an unwholesome or unbalanced diet, they cause many ailments in their babies. For example, a diet excessive in one humor will slowly alter the quality of milk, and the baby will have that humor vitiated. Human milk has been used as a medicine to cure eye and nose ailments, and mild hemorrhages.

Milk products: When fresh milk is boiled and then cooled, there is milk skin along with a creamy layer on the top of it. This is heavy to digest and people with low digestive fire should avoid it. It balances *pitta* and *vāta* and is an aphrodisiac.

By adding a little lemon juice to the boiling milk, the milk solids are separated. These solids are very nourishing and easy to digest. They are called *chenā*. *Chenā* is separated from the liquid by filtering it through a thin cotton cloth. *Chenā* is easy to digest and is used to prepare many salty and sweet dishes. The remaining liquid from this preparation is strength-promoting and is recommended for weak people who have a low power of digestion.

Yogurt: Pure yogurt, called curd in India, is made by adding bacterial cultures of *Lactobacillus* or *streptococcus* species to fresh milk. (You can add a spoon of yogurt with an active culture in it from the health food store; see recipe on page 48.) These bacteria grow very fast in the milk at an appropriate temperature (around 99° F) and make the milk coagulate. In the West, there are many varieties of commercial yogurts which are generally prepared by adding starches, fruits, flavors and/or preservatives. With these varied preparations, sometimes the bacterial culture of the yogurt is dead. What is important is that you should eat a yogurt which has a living culture of bacteria. I recommend highly that you make your own yogurt. A simple method is described later. For making sweet yogurts, you may add marmalade, fruit jams, or even fresh fruits, honey, etc. in the prepared yogurt.

Freshly prepared yogurt should be used right away. Some people may not be able to make yogurt at home due to time constraints. In that case, it is recommended to get fresh, plain yogurt with living bacteria from the health food stores. Avoid buying yogurts that have a long conservation time. Do not buy yogurt when it is close to the expiration date, as it tends to turn sour. When kept for a long time, yogurt turns sour and vitiates the humors.

Fresh yogurt is sweet and highly strength-giving. It promotes *pitta* and *kapha* and cures vitiated *vāta*. It is especially recommended for curing stomach ailments and increasing potency. Yogurt should be eaten in the morning or at noon, but not at night. Excessive intake of yogurt may lead to excess of *pitta* and related disorders.

Yogurt drinks, or *lassī*, are made by whipping yogurt and then adding three times more water in it. It may be made sweet or salty. (See the recipe on page 59.) Sweet *lassī* is *kapha*-promoting and it brings down *pitta*. Salty *lassī* is made by adding some rock salt, cumin powder, and pepper. This drink is good for *vāta*-dominating people.

EGGS

The present book essentially deals with Āyurvedic vegetarian foods and cooking as I, myself, was born and brought up in this tradition. Our familial tradition of not eating any animal products that involve pain and killing (we do use milk, milk products, and eggs) is probably more than 2000 years old. Therefore, I am not the appropriate person to write about non-vegetarian recipes and neither do I recommend them from a personal point of view. However, Āyurveda deals extensively with animal products. It is said that due to geographical locations (in the remote hill areas), or due to emergency situations (war, drought, famine, etc.), human beings may need to eat meat. Āyurveda, as a scientific discipline, takes a neutral stand, and describes the intrinsic qualities of all foods available in nature.

Chicken eggs are *pitta*-promoting and decrease *vāta*. They are strength-giving and have an aphrodisiac effect. These are prescribed to women who have problems related to embryo transplantation. Because of their *pitta*-promoting qualities, eggs should be eaten in moderate quantities, and should be prepared with ghee and vegetables.

Fish eggs are also *pitta*-promoting, and are an aphrodisiac.

HERBS AND SPICES

We will discuss the Āyurvedic properties of certain selected herbs and spices so you may learn their appropriate use for preparing a wholesome meal. Herbs and spices play a very important part in Āyurvedic nutrition. They are strong in their Āyurvedic properties, and are used for bringing humoral equilibrium in food. They enhance the taste and flavor of the food and render it more appetizing. Spices and herbs are generally very rich in minerals and vitamins, and provide additional supplements. They also facilitate digestion and safeguard us from internal disorders. For example, the addition of ginger renders rich and heavy food lighter and easier to digest. However, spices and herbs should be used wisely, according to the specific need, and in an appropriate quantity. Some people think that the use of spices make food very "hot,"

Special Ingredients

Because there is a large population of emigrants from the Indian continent in English-speaking countries, many Indian grocery shops will cater to your needs. In the metropolitan areas, you will find a number of these shops. The shops may even order certain items for clients. I have given many names in Hindi so that readers can write to these shops to ask for the appropriate products. Readers are requested to verify products with the detailed descriptions which I have given, and the Hindi names, which are usually written on the packets sold in these shops. The English translations may sometimes be incorrect. For example, *kalongi*, which has nothing in common with cumin, or any of its varieties, is sometimes translated as black cumin in the USA. There is a variety of cumin known in Hindi as *kala jira*, literally meaning "black cumin." Similarly, *Urad dal* is translated as black gram in some books and I have also used this translation here. But this may be confused with the black beans from Spain. A smaller and dark brown variety of chickpeas is also called *kala channa* in Hindi, literally meaning black chickpeas. Thus, to avoid confusion, verify the name in Hindi and also see the description given in this book. Ghee is also available in these shops, but it is very simple to make (see page 47). Since it can be preserved, one may make a quantity that will last for six months.

The names and addresses of these shops may be found in local telephone directories. In remote areas, one should try to order by mail. According to my experience, in smaller towns, Indian foods may be supplied by Oriental, Turkish, Egyptian, or Indonesian stores. Many of the products mentioned here are also available at health food stores. For example, most of the spices, some exotic vegetables and fruits, fresh full cream milk, yogurt with living culture, different kinds of flours and grains, are sold to health-conscious people.

Sometimes, seed shops may be able to provide you with some of the ingredients for spices. Cardamom (both big and small), cloves, cinnamon, and other spices which are popular for their medicinal value are also kept by pharmacists, apothecaries, or drug stores. In some places, herb shops are another source where one can buy products like licorice, ajwain, long pepper, etc.

and they are unable to eat hot food. They confuse spices with red or green hot chilies.

You should make sure that the spices you buy are fresh. Old spices lose their taste, flavor, and pharmacological properties. Do not buy powdered spices. Make your own powders a little before use. That may be done with a small stone, metal mortar, or an electric grinder, like the coffee grinder.

Many of the spices described below are available in supermarkets or in the health food stores in the West. In most European and American cities, there are Indian or Pakistani food stores that cater to the needs of Indians who live here. You may find the addresses of these shops in your local telephone book. Let us now learn about the properties of some important spices for their appropriate use.

Ajwain *(Trachyspermum ammi)*: This will probably only be available in Indian food stores. These are tiny, light brown seeds. They have a pungent taste and a flavor which resembles thyme. Ajwain increases *pitta* and cures vitiated *kapha* and *vāta*.

Anise *(Funiculum vulgare)*: Anise seeds cure vitiated *vāta* and *pitta*, and promote digestion. They are eaten after meals for perfuming the mouth and getting rid of the flavor of strong spices.

Black pepper *(Piper nigrum)*: Black pepper cures vitiated *vāta* and *kapha* and increases *pitta*. There is also another variety which is white. This is prepared from black pepper by removing the black skin with special methods. Both have the same properties.

Cardamom *(Elettaria cardamomum)*: Cardamom has an exclusive flavor and is used to perfume both sweet and salty food. Cardamom seeds are dark brown to blackish and are in light green pods. Outside India, there is also a variety available with white pods, but it has different taste and qualities. Peel the pods just before use and crush the seeds. Cardamom brings an equilibrium to the humors and promotes digestion. Besides using it in food, it is highly recommended to chew cardamom after meals. This helps remove the strong flavor of some substances like garlic, fenugreek, etc.

Cardamom, Greater *(Amomum subulatum)*: In pods like the cardamom, but the pods are three to four times bigger in size and

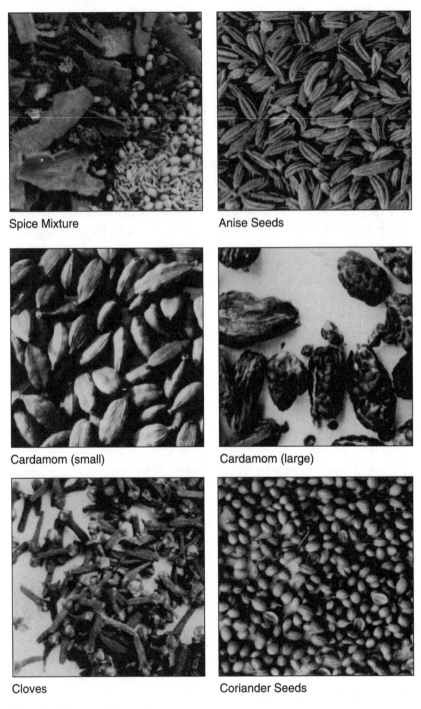

Spice Mixture

Anise Seeds

Cardamom (small)

Cardamom (large)

Cloves

Coriander Seeds

Figure 3. Close-ups of some spices.

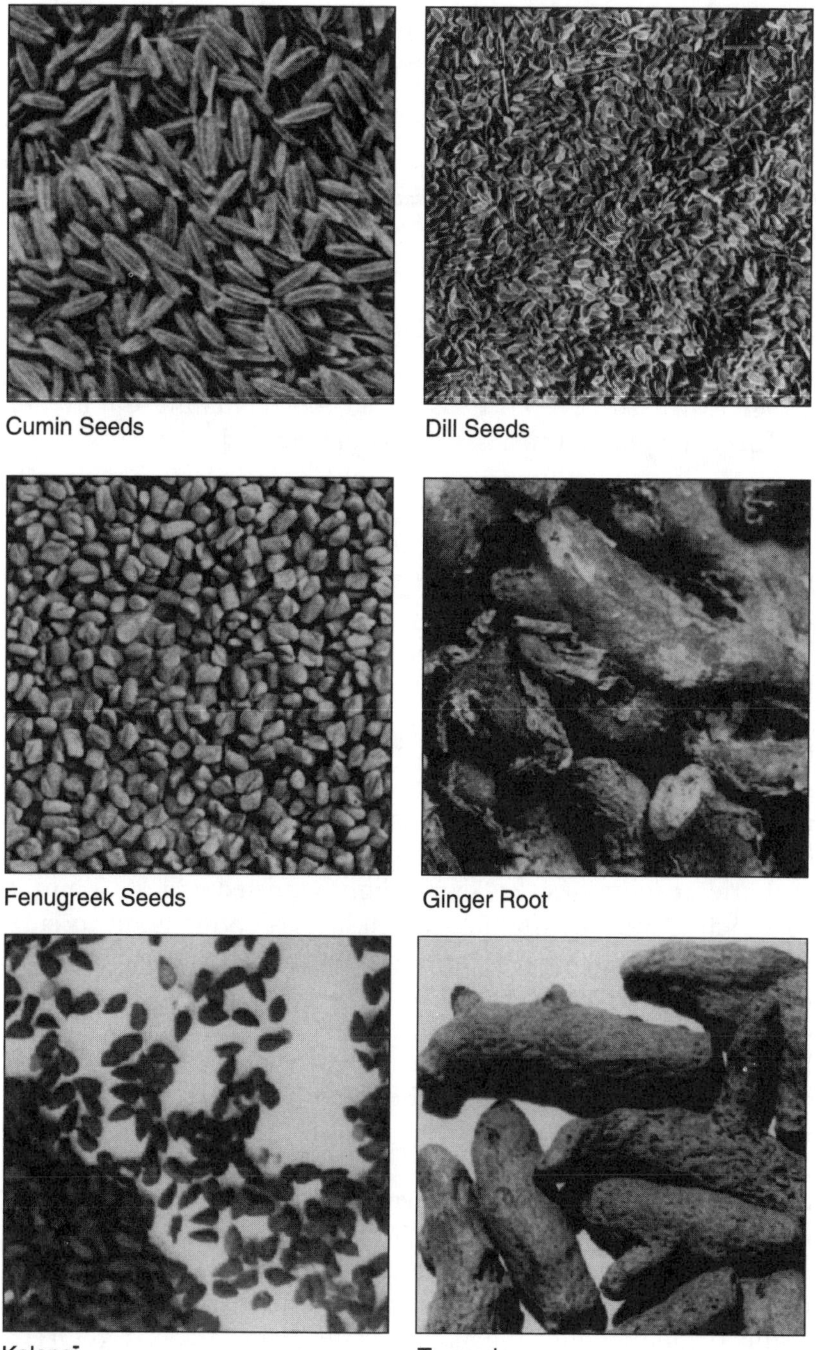

Cumin Seeds

Dill Seeds

Fenugreek Seeds

Ginger Root

Kalongī

Turmeric

Figure 4. Close-ups of some spices.

are brown. The seeds are dark brown. Despite the similarity in the name, the taste and properties of the greater cardamom are different from regular cardamom. It cures vitiated *vata* and *kapha*, but increases *pitta*.

Cinnamon *(Cinnamomum zeylanicum):* The part used is the bark. Cinnamon is used frequently in Western cuisine now. It cures vitiated *vata* and *kapha*, but it increases *pitta*.

Clove *(Syzygium aeromaticum):* Cloves are brown and look like little buds. They are dried buds. They are highly perfumed and pungent in taste. They are also used for perfuming the mouth and are chewed after meals. Cloves cure vitiated *pitta* and *kapha*.

Coriander *(Coriandur sativum):* Coriander seeds and leaves are used. You may grow some seeds in pots to get fresh leaves used to flavor salads as well as vegetable preparations. The leaves should not be cooked, as they lose their flavor upon heating. Seeds are roundish in shape, and yellow in color. Coriander cures vitiated humors, especially vitiated *pitta*.

Cumin *(Cuminum cyminum):* There are several varieties sold under this name. The light brown cumin seeds with straight edges are good for cooking. The two other varieties available are also called carvi or caraway, are darker in color, and smaller in size, and one of them has seeds with slightly turned edges. Cumin is very rich in various vitamins and minerals and is good to cure weakness and fatigue. It promotes digestion. It cures vitiated *vata* and *kapha*, and enhances *pitta*.

Dill *(Anethum sowa):* Dill leaves cure vitiated *kapha* and *vata*. However, the more effective part is the seeds. But generally leaves are used as an herb.

Fenugreek *(Trigonella foenumgraecum):* This spice is lesser known abroad. However, it is available in health food stores. The seeds are used as spice, and the leaves are used in salads or as vegetables. Fenugreek is very good to cure vitiated *vata* and its use is highly recommended. You may grow the seeds in pots to get fresh leaves to use as a winter vegetable.

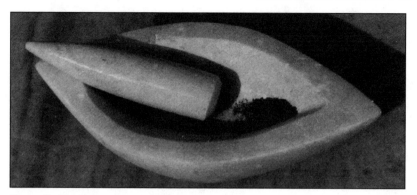

Figure 5. Marble mortar with kalongī inside.

Garlic *(Allium sativum)*: Fresh garlic cures vitiated *vāta* and *kapha*, but enhances *pitta*. Therefore, you should not use garlic with *pitta*-promoting substances. You should use a moderate quantity of garlic as its excessive use gives rise to too much thirst and restlessness. Daily, moderate use of garlic is highly recommended.

Ginger *(Gingiber officinale)*: These days, fresh ginger is available nearly everywhere. It is available in big stores, Indian, Chinese, or Turkish shops, or health food stores. Ginger is a great appetizer and promotes digestive power. It cures vitiated *vāta* and *kapha*.

Kalongī *(Nigella sativa)*: These are black, tiny seeds with one side round and the other side conical. Kalongī cures vitiated *vāta* and *kapha*, but enhances *pitta*. It is available at Indian food stores. Sometimes, it is erroneously called black cumin.

Mustard *(Brassica campestris)*: Mustard seeds are used as a spice, and their paste is used in salad dressings. Mustard seeds cure *vāta* and *kapha*, but increase *pitta*. They should not be used in excess.

Turmeric *(Curcuma, longa)*: This is a root like ginger, but is yellow in color. It is that which gives the yellow color in so called "curry" in the West. "Curry" is a mixture of many spices that includes Curcuma or turmeric. But in India, we do not use spices in such a non-specific way. It is better to make one's own mixtures and watch the proportions of each ingredient one uses. Turmeric is

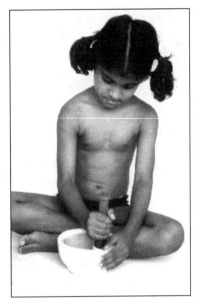

Figure 6. Clay mortar.

sold mostly in powder form as it is very hard to crush. You should
make sure that it is not too old, and it should have its characteris-
tic strong smell. Turmeric cures vitiated humors and provides
color and flavor to vegetables.

BEVERAGES, OILS, SWEETENERS

It is important to understand the Āyurvedic properties of some
other frequently used substances such as cooking oils, sugars,
juices, tea and coffee, and alcoholic beverages.

Alcoholic beverages: The use of old wine in moderate quantity,
with food, is recommended in Āyurveda. It purifies the body,
cures vitiated *vāta* and *kapha*, and is good for the digestive fire.
However, new wines vitiate humors, are heavy, and cause indigestion. Wine or other alcoholic beverages should be taken in very

moderate quantity, with or after food, only when one is healthy and does not feel depressed. When alcoholic beverages are taken in excess, they bring down the body's *ojas* (energy and immunity) and one becomes vulnerable to ailments and diseases.

Cold drinks: These days, many carbonated cold drinks are sold all over the world. The use of carbonated water is also very frequent. It is better to use plain water. Cold drinks have a high sugar content, sweeteners, or other chemicals, and should be avoided. Some have caffeine which produces nervousness and insomnia.

Fruit juices: According to Āyurveda, only freshly pressed juices should be used. The use of previously pressed juices enhances *vāta*.

Honey: The properties of honey depend largely upon its source, the flowers the bees used to make it. Generally, honey is good for vision and cures vitiated *kapha*. According to Āyurveda, honey is an antagonist to heat, and therefore should not be used in hot preparations. If taken hot, it vitiates all the humors.

Oils: The use of oil in cooking and food preparation is essential, as it controls the excess *vāta*. Oils are *pitta*-promoting and are essential for the metabolizing of certain substances in our food. The use of vegetable oils is absolutely essential for having healthy and beautiful skin. According to Āyurveda, sesame oil is the best of all the oils available. These days, the use of groundnut oil, sunflower oil, and corn oil is also frequent. Coconut and corn oil do not enhance *pitta*, but they increase *kapha*. Olive oil, like sesame oil, is very good for the skin and promotes appetite. Do not buy mixed vegetable oils, as they may contain cheap oils, like rapeseed oil, which is harmful for health and vitiates all three humors.

Sugar: The use of sugar has increased tremendously in the West after the Second World War. It is mostly eaten in the form of sweets, chocolates, and bakery products. White crystal sugar should be avoided. Cane sugar products are better among the various sugar preparations. The use of candy sugar and brown sugar is recommended. Sugar cures vitiated *vāta* and *pitta*, but it enhances *kapha*. Candy sugar is an exception; it does not increase *kapha*.

Tea and coffee: Both tea and coffee are popular all over the world. They are "hot" in their Āyurvedic properties. They are *vāta*-decreasing, anti-fatigue and anti-sleep. Too much tea gives rise to stomach acidity and vitiates *pitta*. Excessive use of coffee gives rise to chest pain, nervousness, and insomnia.

OUR RELATIONSHIP TO FOOD

First of all, you learned about the basic constitution with respect to the three humors. Then you learned that our environment changes our humoral equilibrium, and that the key to good health is to live with the rhythm of the changes taking place in nature. Third, you learned about the Āyurvedic qualities of various foods. Now I will discuss coordinating the humoral qualities of various foods with the humoral nature so you can maintain a humoral balance. This, however, does not mean that you should mathematically eat foods that have certain humoral qualities you require, while avoiding foods that enhance your dominating humor. It is important to learn to prepare combinations that are wholesome. There is no doubt that naturally wholesome foods are good for health and are easy to digest. But you cannot limit yourself to only certain foods. The joy of the palate is also essential in life. Healthy food should not mean insipid food.

Āyurveda does not propose that foods are healthy or unhealthy. Nutrition is allied to various factors like weather, climate, place, time, and your humoral composition. Therefore, it is important to learn to prepare wholesome food, to eat in a wholesome way (with respect to quality, quantity, and the way you eat) and according to place and time. It is observed that many health fanatics eat insipid food and many of them very strongly propagate vegetarianism. According to the concepts of Āyurveda, the food should always be a delight to the palate besides being wholesome. One should not ignore sensory pleasures and delights in life. However, the senses should not be uncontrolled; meaning, thereby, that if the food is delicious, you should not prolong that sensory pleasure and fall ill or get fat. This is an essential and very important message. Enjoy all aspects of sensuality but always govern your actions, and have an appropriate control of your mind over your senses.

Quality and Quantity of Food

If you saturate yourself excessively with unctuous, sweet, heavy, slimy substances, or new cereals, fresh wine, milk and its products, sugar and flour preparations, and abstain from physical movement; if you use comfortable seats and beds, sleep during the day; suffer from diseases caused by over-saturation, if not counteracted promptly,[3] it is said that you may also suffer from diabetes, itching, anemia, fever, lassitude, heaviness in the body, obstruction in sense organs and channels, disorders of the mind, drowsiness, and all kinds of digestive orders.

> One having regular physical exercise, taking food only after the previous meal is digested, eating barley and wheat, does not suffer from obesity and is relieved of the disorders caused by over-saturation. The remedy for the disorders caused by over-saturation is under-nutritional regiment.[4]

On the contrary to over-saturation, some people eat less than their requirements, they have a loss of appetite or other digestive troubles, or they may develop an aversion to food due to mental problems, such as depression. If they ignore their problems over a long period of time, they become victims of many ailments.

> Loss of body weight, digestive power, strength, luster, sexual excretions and musculature, fever, continuous cough, weakness in hearing, insanity, delirium, cardiac pain, obstruction of urine and stool, pain in shanks, thighs and sacral region, pain in joints, and other *vāta* disorders, like the upward movements of wind, etc., are caused by under-nutrition. They are treated by experts with saturating measures which may exhibit their effect instantly or after a prolonged use.[5]

> Food or any other thing that is unwholesome and that has unpleasant consequences should not be used out of ignorance or carelessness. . . . One should eat warm, unctuous food, in proper quantity, after the previous food is digested, non-antagonistic, in a favorable place with all the favorable accessories, not too fast, not too slow, not

---

[3] *Caraka Saṃhitā, Sūtrasthāna*, XXIII, 3–5.
[4] *Caraka Saṃhitā, Sūtrasthāna*, XXIII, 25.
[5] *Caraka Saṃhitā, Sūtrasthāna*, XXIII, 27–30.

while talking or laughing, with full concentration, and after due consideration to the self.[6]

Some of the statements quoted above need explanations. It is recommended to take warm and unctuous food. Cold, rough, and dry food enhances *vāta* and is not good in our times when we have enough *vāta*-enhancing factors because of our food technology and the hectic pace of life. ". . . Warm food stimulates the digestive fire, gets digested quickly, has a carminative effect on flatus and reduces mucous."[7] Thus, eating cold dinners will be against Āyurvedic instructions. A *vāta*-increasing diet may not have an immediate effect during our youth, but it will have a long term ill effect. We know that old age is *vāta*-dominating, and in addition to that, if we are eating *vāta*-dominated food, we may endanger ourselves for *vāta* ailments, and various pains and aches, gout, or arthritis may develop later in life. This means we should reconsider eating salads for our night meal in the winter, especially in cold countries.

Unctuous food means food with fat. Some quantity of fat is absolutely essential for digestion and assimilation. Certain vitamins are not assimilated in the body without the presence of fat. That is why the most traditional methods of making salad include oil, or salads are eaten with other foods containing fat.

Both animal and plant fats are essential for us. One gets animal fat from butter, and plant fat from vegetable oils, nuts, and so on. Small amounts of both animal and plant fat can be included in the meals.

Āyurveda gives precise instructions on the quantity of food one should consume. It is true that the quantity of food varies from person to person, according to the power of digestion, age, weight, etc. However, there is a general principle one should follow: never eat to saturation. One should only fill two thirds of the stomach with solids and liquids. One third of the stomach should be left empty for the three humors. If the stomach is completely filled, then there is no place left for the humors, and they are pushed up, causing discomfort and giving rise to several ailments related to digestion. It is recommended not to take liquids or

---

[6] *Caraka Saṃhitā, Vimānasthānam*, I, 23–24.
[7] *Caraka Saṃhitā, Vimānasthānam*, I, 24 (1).

water with foods, so the stomach does not get full very quickly. It is recommended to drink water one hour after the meal. According to the Āyurvedic tradition, it is not wise to take juices, milk, or other liquids with the main meal. Soups are recommended. A light yogurt drink *(lassī)* may be taken in summer. It is suggested to take some old wine in the traditional texts of Āyurveda. In any case, one should not fill one's stomach more than two thirds with either solids or liquids.

The quantity of food should also be decided according to the quality of the food one is taking. Some substances are easy to digest, whereas others are heavy and hard to digest. Pulses, lentils, and some grains are heavy to digest, and green leafy vegetables are lighter. Rice is lighter to digest than wheat, and corn is heavier than wheat. These are some examples to help you determine the quantity you should consume. Heavy substances, if taken in a small quantity, become light, whereas light substances become heavy if taken in a large quantity. Thus, quantity is one of the factors determining the heaviness and lightness of the substances. You may take a light substance up to the point of saturation, but a heavy substance should be taken in small quantity.

You should eat only after the previous meal is completely digested. Sometimes people eat because it is mealtime, and not that they are really hungry. This should not be done, as the fresh food gets mixed with the half-digested food and the digestive juices, and this vitiates all the humors. This may cause flatus, fermentation, and may diminish the power of digestion.

You should avoid eating between meals, and you should not go for long intervals without any food. Keeping hungry enhances *vāta*. It is better to eat some fruit or something light if your meals are delayed. It is recommended to eat in smaller quantities four times a day, rather than eating only two principal meals.

I have already given Āyurvedic instructions on the quantity of food in relation to the capacity of the stomach. The problem in affluent nations is that people eat too much, which is the root cause of many prevalent disorders. It is the other side of malnutrition compared to the one caused by the scarcity of food. People eat too much, and they do not eat according to their age and activities. Then they suffer from overweight and go to "fitness centers." All this sounds ironic. Learn to have an appropriate control over your senses. Do not eat excessive protein foods when you are an adult. For example, take either cheese, eggs, or some beans containing protein instead of having two or three of these. Eat a light evening meal with some soup and salad, or other vegetable preparations. You may take some cheese if you are not saturated with the above-mentioned products. Always include fruits in your meals. As you have read earlier, beef and potatoes are unwholesome foods. Do not eat an excess of any of these, and try to eat a variety of foods instead of repeatedly eating the same things. Incorporate rice in your meals to replace bread from time to time, as rice is a lighter food than wheat. The recipes on the following pages may inspire you to eat a different variety of foods.

If you wish to decrease the quantity of food you consume, do this very slowly. Actually, gradually people begin to eat too much and their digestive fire *(agni)* goes on increasing. You have to do the reverse of that by slowly cutting down on the quantity, as well as by changing from heavy food to lighter food. For example, you may eat more rice or fruits or some other light foodstuff. By eating too much, people lose their joy of life, and live constantly under the fear of getting fat, or they suffer from various disorders caused by obesity.

Antagonism in Food

Certain combinations of foods should never be taken because of their opposite nature. Various foods can be antagonistic to each other, or to the time, place, or state of a person. For example, yogurt or curd should be taken in the morning with breakfast and at noon with lunch, but should not be eaten for dinner. If at all, one should take it with cumin, pepper, and some ghee. Sweet curd should not be eaten at night. "One fond of curd and using it recklessly suffers from fever, internal hemorrhage, anemia, giddiness and jaundice."[8]

Nuts should not be eaten in the summer, as they promote *pitta.* Your diet should be based on the place where you live. In cold places, you need a *pitta*-dominating diet, whereas in arid and hot lands, you need more sweets and a liquid diet, such as sweet cold drinks, cold milk, the juices of sweet fruits, and light meals in

---

[8] *Caraka Saṃhitā, Sūtrasthāna,* VII, 62.

ANTAGONISM IN FOOD

Antagonists are substances, actions, or preparations that react contrary to the nature of the body. The antagonism may be caused by the food itself, by various food combinations, processing, place, time, dose, etc. When antagonistic substances are eaten, one subjects oneself to various forms of antagonism in reference to the Āyurvedic instructions. Antagonistic foods produce terrible effects. Sometimes, the effect may take the form of an immediate malaise, whereas at other times a slow effect may take place. In this latter case, the antagonism may lead to a serious disease. Minor ailments due to antagonisms in food give rise to chronic ailments. Therefore, you should be selective when combining foods. Eating antagonistic food is like giving yourself a slow dose of poison. The following list mentions some common antagonists:

1. Milk with water melon.
2. Milk with radishes.
3. Milk with sour things.
4. Honey with wine.
5. Honey in hot drinks.
6. Hot water after taking honey.
7. Cold after intake of ghee or other oily substance.
8. Sweet and cold food eaten by a person accustomed to pungent and hot, or vice versa.
9. Use of diet, drug, behavior adverse to a person's practice.
10. Antagonism in processing, such as the use of food technology which may render food unsuitable.
11. Antagonism from cooking, such as cooking with bad fuel, uncooked, over-cooked, or burned food.
12. Not eating according to seasons, such as eating nuts in summer, cold drinks in winter, etc.
13. Eating yogurt at night.
14. Drinking something too hot or too cold.
15. Combinations of hot and cold.
16. Intake of too salty, sharp, pungent, or sour substances.
17. Not eating according to the geographic location, such as eating rough and sharp in arid zones.
18. Intake of *vāta*-vitiating substances by a person indulging in overwork, sexual intercourse, or physical exercise.
19. *Kapha*-vitiating substances by a person indulging in excessive sleep and laziness.
20. Not eating according to one's constitution.

general. Certain foods are antagonistic in combination. There are others that are antagonistic in certain forms, like honey in a hot drink. Pre-prepared foods *(bāsā)* and pre-pressed juices are *vāta*-promoting, and they are antagonistic in respect to the humors. For details of antagonists, see page 41.

Āyurveda does not recommend that you eat old or dry foods. Bread which is not freshly made is a dry and old food. Do not buy breads which can be preserved for a week or more. Preferably, make your own fresh breads or crêpes as described on the following pages. All preserved food is not recommended, whether it is canned or frozen. Similarly, fruit juices which are preserved are very harmful and give rise to *vāta*-related disorders. It is recommended to take water or a small quantity of old wine with main meals instead of preserved juices. If you wish to drink a fruit juice, make it yourself and consume it immediately. Otherwise, eat fresh fruits. Similarly, avoid milk which is processed to keep for a long time. Make your own yogurt and ghee. Eat simple and little, but well. Food technology in the West is very advanced, and has evolved various methods to preserve foodstuffs for a very long time. This opens the way to more inborn disorders.

Try to buy pure products that are not prepared, that do not contain chemical preservatives. Do not use products with sodium glutamate or other taste-enhancing chemicals. Do not buy salty foods, such as salted nuts. Try to buy them in natural conditions. You may add salt yourself if you like. Then you can have a control on the quantity you are adding.

Food Consumption

Besides the appropriate quality and quantity of food, the surroundings and the aesthetic appeal of the presentation of the food is also important. Sit in a comfortable posture in pleasant surroundings. It is recommended to sit cross-legged when eating food, but many Westerners cannot sit comfortably in this posture. Whatever way you sit, do not sit in an odd posture, or stand and eat. In a standing posture, the stomach and intestines are not completely relaxed and the food is not digested well.

The presentation of food is equally important. It should be nicely served in appropriate utensils. Delicious food served on plastic or paper plates kills its taste and intrinsic value, and makes it look uninspiring. It is a pity that the American practice of fast food, where one stands and eats, or the food is served in paper and Styrofoam utensils, is spreading all over the world. I remember that when I went to the United States for the first time in 1979, American food culture was a great shock to me. Having lived in India and France, where food is so important, and so much time, money, and energy is devoted to it, the United States was a great contrast, for it seemed that people ate just to keep alive and not for joy. This was a great surprise to me.

Before beginning to eat, one should bring oneself mentally to the process of eating. One should not "jump on food" and devour it. Wash your hands before sitting for a meal, and say something like this before beginning to eat: "May this food bring me energy and vigor, keep me healthy and make me live long. May this food keep the humors in balance. I am grateful to Mother Earth, the water, the Sun, the wind, and the ether, for providing me with this food." You may make your own text in whatever way you wish. The important thing is to attain consciousness about the eating process, coming to the realization that food is life-giving, and a very important part of our being.

Food should not be eaten too quickly or too slowly, and should be chewed properly. Eating too quickly or too slowly will enhance *vāta*. One should relish food and try to distinguish the diverse tastes in it. This will enhance the sense of taste, which is not only good for sensory pleasure, but also helps to detect any spoiled, harmful, or old food, and will save one from any kind of food poisoning.

In the above quotation from Caraka, it is written that one should not eat while talking or laughing. It does not mean that long dinners with many courses and conversation, as in French homes, are forbidden in Āyurveda. It specifically means that during the process of chewing, one should not talk or laugh, as this can cause obstruction in the wind pipe.

Do not eat when you are afflicted with emotions like passion, anger, greed, confusion, envy, grief, conceit, excitement, or fear. Always calm down before eating. I have often heard at home that the food taken in a state of anger or depression becomes poisonous when inside the body. Eating during emotional stress gives rise to gas, flatus, stiffness of the intestines, and other gastric troubles. If it is done frequently and over a period of time, it leads to stomach ulcers.

It is said that one should eat "after a due consideration to the self." It means that one should always eat keeping in mind what is good for oneself. Even when the food is delicious and one is tempted, one should keep in mind the things which are not suitable to oneself according to one's Āyurvedic nature (humoral composition). For example, if you know that cabbage does not suit you, and you get stomach problems from it, or if a certain variety of cheese gives you blisters in the mouth, and so on, you should not eat these, despite the fact that you like them and you are tempted. One should not invite trouble. In addition, you should not try things that do not suit you. Perhaps they are harmless when you eat them in small quantities. Therefore, realize your limits and also learn varied preparation methods to make the foods wholesome.

BEING A VEGETARIAN

Twenty-four years ago, when I went to France as a student, my newly made friends were horrified by my peculiar habits of not eating meat and fish. Inviting me for a meal was a real problem for them. I was unable to convince them that the delicious cheese of their country, and the bread and salads made a sufficient meal for me. They felt embarrassed to invite me, and I must admit that after the spicy meals of my homeland, the boiled vegetables tasted awful to my tongue. On the other hand, when I invited these friends for food, they were very apprehensive of a vegetarian meal: "I did not know that one can eat so well being a vegetarian," or "Is this meal really without meat? We did not feel its absence." Another apprehension people had was that vegetarians are physically weak persons. I often had to remind them that elephants are vegetarians.

In the late 1970s, the era of macrobiotic and vegetarian food shops and restaurants came to Paris, and other cities of Western Europe. I moved to the U.S. in 1980, where vegetarianism was widespread, and people often asked me, "Since when are you a vegetarian?" I had no answer to this question, as I had not known otherwise. This seems to be our familial way since eternity.

Whether you are a vegetarian or not, to keep good health and have a long life, it is important to eat a wholesome diet. Regular meals should be consumed in an appropriate manner and in moderate quantity. Your food should be fresh, of good quality, well-prepared, and tasty. People who eat meat should realize that meat alone can never make a wholesome diet, and it should not be consumed in excess. From time to time I came across people in Europe who ate meat or fish products two to three times a day, and they ate very little grain or vegetables. This is an investment in disaster for the later part of one's life.

If someone wants to convert from eating meat to vegetarian food, one needs not remain either undernourished or eat insipid food. One should make this transition slowly, and with appropriate knowledge about selecting ingredients and preparing food. A vegetarian meal cooked without suitable spices and other ingredients may lead to a serious deficiency of minerals and vitamins. Meat is relatively easy to prepare, whereas vegetables need skill in their preparation. Meat is a comprehensive food, whereas a vegetarian diet needs a larger variety of combinations to make a complete meal. However, one cannot make a complete diet with only meat products. A regular consumption of cereals, vegetables, and other plant products is absolutely essential. One can make a vegetarian diet complete and wholesome, but it is most important to learn that a vegetarian diet is also incomplete and unwholesome without animal products. The animal products consumed by vegetarians are dairy products, such as milk, butter, ghee, cheese, yogurt, etc. I know that some people in Europe and in the U.S. are vegetarians in the sense of eating only plant products, and they strictly avoid butter, cheese, or eggs. Āyurveda does not recommend that. I do not suggest that anyone should take to the vegan kind of vegetarianism. It may open doors for ill health due to malnutrition, and may give rise to incurable disorders. In any case, one should not go to any extreme, or become fanatic, in the process of maintaining good health. Fanaticism never gives rise to balance and harmony, and in Āyurveda, balance is the principle that forms the basis for good health. In any case, whether you wish to eat meat or not, always eat good quality food.

You have already learned about the Āyurvedic nature of varied foodstuffs and the characteristics of the spices. On the following pages, I have provided some preparation methods for a wholesome diet. These will allow you to be "a vegetarian without suffering," and you will not miss your good old meat-eating days. The important thing is that you should not be lazy in preparing and shopping, and you should always keep a few things in stock. For example, you should have at least two or three kinds of different flours, various grains and spices, onions, ginger, garlic, rice, milk yogurt, cooking oil, and ghee. You need to buy a variety of fresh vegetables and fruits, but it is not essential to do this every day. In case you are unable to shop sometimes, with the help of the above ingredients, a small but tasty meal can be prepared.

3

PREPARING FOODS

THE RECIPES THAT follow in this chapter are not classic recipes. They are based upon Āyurvedic principles and are recipes that I have made. When I mention well-known foods, such as *dāls*, *chapātī*, etc., I have used the common names for the dishes. However, most of the books on Āyurvedic cooking are simply Indian cookbooks. All Indian cooking is not Āyurvedic, and Āyurvedic cooking does not have to be Indian style. I feel that food combining is the most important concept that you can learn.

I have already discussed the qualities of food products and our relationship to food in general. The following simple methods of food preparation will help you use various spices for making wholesome meals that provide the body a humoral equilibrium and a feeling of well-being. I do not suggest that you change your food habits entirely, but hope that you become aware of the possibilities of a wholesome diet.

BASIC PREPARATIONS

After describing some fundamental preparations, such as ghee, yogurt, mixtures of spices, etc., I will continue with some recipes for breakfast, preparing bread from different grains, and some rice preparations. This will be continued with methods for preparing dāls (lentils), vegetables, eggs, desserts, and some drinks.

Ghee or Clarified Butter

Butter is not 100 percent fat. The process of making ghee involves eliminating all the other components and keeping the pure fat.

Ghee has a different flavor than butter, and can be preserved for many years. Ghee is a very healthy fat for cooking, and it renders a delicate taste and flavor to food. Do not buy readymade butter fat, as it contains preservatives. Ghee made at home does not require anything to preserve it.

For making ghee, take pure, unsalted butter, put it in a pot and melt it on a low fire. Let it cook until you see a clear transparent liquid and some residue around and on the bottom of the pot. Stir it from time to time while it is cooking. Take care that it does not turn brown. The cooking time depends upon the intensity of the fire (stove temperature) and the quality of butter. After it is ready, let it cool a little, and then filter it through a muslin cloth while it is still warm, in order to remove the residue. Store the ghee in dry, clean, and tightly closed bottles. Ghee has a semisolid consistency, and is a light yellow color when it's cool. However, at warmer temperatures, ghee becomes transparent and looks like other cooking oils.

Yogurt

For making yogurt, first boil commercial full cream milk. Put the milk in an earthen vessel which can retain heat for a long time. When the milk cools down to a temperature which is not unpleasantly hot to your fingers, add ½ teaspoon plain yogurt with active bacteria in it, and mix it well with the milk. Put a lid on the pot and cover it well from all sides with a small blanket or an old woolen pullover so that it keeps warm. Keep it in a warm place for 8 to 10 hours, or overnight. This yogurt can be preserved in your refrigerator for 3–4 days.

Spice Mixtures

I will describe below two principal spice mixtures which may be used in various preparations for attaining humoral balance, as a supplement of minerals and vitamins, and for facilitating digestion. The first mixture is prepared by grinding six different spices and is generally known as *garam masālā* in northwestern India. I do not recommend buying a readymade mixture because the quality and proportion of the spices is not as good as when it is made at home. For making this mixture, combine ¼ cup of each of the following: cumin, greater cardamom, cloves, cinnamon, nutmeg, and black pepper. Add ½ cup coriander. Clean each of the spices well. Take the greater cardamom out of the pods. Mix all the spices. Dry them for a day or two in a warm dry place (in the sun or in a heated room). Grind all these spices in a mortar or a grinder, and mix well the powder obtained. A small grinder, which is generally used for grinding coffee beans may be bought for the spices. Do not grind the spices into a very fine powder; keep them like grains of sand. Store the mixture in tightly closed, preferably dark glass bottles. This mixture can be kept for a year. For your convenience, I call this Spice Mixture A for all further references.

The second mixture is made with an equal quantity of kalongī, anise, cumin, fenugreek, and mustard seeds. Each of them should be cleaned, mixed well, and kept unground in tightly closed bottles. We call this Spice Mixture B for all further references.

Sprouts

According to various texts of Āyurveda, the most beneficial and wholesome state of germinating grains is when they are just beginning to germinate. For obtaining this state, it is generally sufficient to keep the grains for 24 to 36 hours in water or a wet muslin cloth. It is recommended to sprout brown chick peas, mung beans, and wheat. Clean and wash the grains and soak them in water. After a few hours, you will see that the grains absorb all the water. The process of germination has already been initiated, and the grains have stored enough water for that. Germinated grains are tender, easy to digest, and wholesome.

For an advanced germination of grains, keep them in a wet cloth after having soaked them overnight in water. Keep sprinkling some water on the cloth from time to time to prevent the seeds from drying. Cress, coriander, and fenugreek seeds may be germinated like this to get fresh green vegetables.

RECIPES FOR BREAKFAST

Wheat Porridge

Clean, wash, and dry some wheat and store it in a jar. You may do the same after sprouting or germinating the wheat for about 24 hours. But this latter requires a long time to dry. Take 2 tablespoons of this wheat and grind it partially in a small coffee grinder a little before use. Fry this wheat in 2 teaspoons of ghee on a low fire, while stirring. (This is called "roasting.") When it is roasted, add half a glass of water to the pan, and keep stirring. After it begins to boil, add 1 glass of milk and cook for 2 to 5 minutes on a low fire. You may add some sugar, raisins, and almonds to it while it is cooking. Wheat porridge is a strength-promoting, wholesome breakfast.

The same recipe may be used for a preparation with semolina instead of crushed wheat.

Carrot Milk

This recipe is like that for Wheat Porridge except that here you use grated carrots instead of partially crushed wheat. For the proportions mentioned above, take 2 or 3 medium-sized finely grated carrots. Cook them a little longer in the ghee than you would the wheat in the above-described recipe. After the carrots are well cooked, add the milk directly. You do not need to add water to this recipe.

Germinated Brown Chickpeas

Highly recommended for breakfast for those who suffer from constipation, headaches, and other minor stomach ailments. It is best to eat 1 or 2 tablespoons of slightly germinated grains (when they are just beginning to sprout). They are soft and taste good. You should chew them well. If you want to cook them, you may either fry them in some ghee or boil them. However, it is best to eat them raw.

Fresh Yogurt

Mix fresh yogurt with fruit and honey as a highly recommended breakfast in the Āyurvedic tradition. It is said that yogurt eaten in the morning is like nectar to the body. However, you should not drink tea or coffee with it because they are antagonistic. You may take your tea or coffee half an hour earlier, or two hours after this breakfast.

BREAD

Bread or rice are eaten as staple foods in most of the world. In the affluent West, these grains are not used as staple foods, and instead, large quantities of high protein and fat rich foods, such as meat, eggs, cream, cheese, etc., are consumed. It is recommended that you incorporate more grains in your meals.

When the word "bread" is used, the reader in the West generally associates it with something made of flour and yeast culture. However, in Āyurveda, an excessive use of yeast is forbidden, and yeast is used in very few bread preparations.

Maize Bread

There are many different ways to prepare maize (corn) flour, but this is a very simple and quick recipe. For making bread to be eaten with vegetable dishes, make a thick batter with flour and water. You may add some milk so that the bread does not stick to the pan. Stir the mixture well. Heat the pan and put a little ghee or oil in it. Put some batter on the hot pan and spread it well with a spoon (as is done for making crepes or pancakes). When it is cooked a little bit, turn it over and add a little more ghee. Cook it on low fire.

One may also make this bread by adding vegetables to it. In a batter made with $1\frac{1}{4}$ cup (250 grams) flour, add a finely chopped medium-sized onion, 2 tomatoes, 1 tablespoon chopped fresh ginger, 1 teaspoon mild paprika, 1 teaspoon Spice Mixture A (page 48), 1 teaspoon ajwain, $\frac{1}{2}$ teaspoon salt and 1 hot green chili or $\frac{1}{4}$ teaspoon of red chili powder. This last ingredient is optional; leave it out if you do not like hot food. Mix all these ingredients in the batter and make the bread the same way as described above.

This recipe can also be used to make breads using various types of millet and barley flours. Finger millet breads are delicious if made by adding vegetables. With some yogurt sauce (*rāyatā*) described on page 58, or with some salad, these breads can make a full meal.

Wheat Bread

There are a variety of breads made from wheat that are mentioned in ancient Āyurvedic literature. They are still prepared today in India. The simplest is a thin, flat bread which is called *chapātī*, which is made fresh for each meal. *Chapātī* is eaten with vegetable preparations and is made without salt. A dough is made with finely ground whole wheat flour and water. The dough for *chapātīs* should be well-kneaded and made about half an hour before the preparation of the *chapātīs*. If the dough is well made, it is easy to make *chapātīs*. Take nearly 1 tablespoon of dough and make a ball of it between your palms. Then flatten it with a rolling pin. Use some flour to prevent it from sticking on the surface while rolling. Roll it as thin as possible. Pick it up carefully to put in the hot pan. No fat is used for making *chapātīs*. Turn it over after a few seconds. Do not have the flame too high (or the electric stove too hot). Turn it over again and then press the surface with a piece of cotton cloth. By doing so, the *chapātī* will puff up. It is ready. Remove it from the pan and make the next one. Put a little bit of ghee on the surface of each *chapātī*. It is a matter of practice: it takes some time until one begins to make *chapātīs* quickly.

Chickpea Flour Bread

This bread is made with a mixture of chickpea flour *(basin)* and whole wheat *chapātī* flour, in a ratio of one to three. Add 1 finely chopped onion, 2 teaspoons finely chopped fresh ginger, 1 green chili (optional), ½ teaspoon each ajwain and salt, and 1 teaspoon Spice Mixture A to 1¼ cups (250 grams) of the flour mixture. Mix all this and make a dough with water, as described above for the *chapātīs*. Take nearly twice as much dough as you took for making a *chapātī*, and flatten it the same way. This bread is not thin like the *chapātīs*. It is cooked in the pan with some ghee like corn bread.

Dosās

This is a kind of thin salty pancake made with rice and black gram flour. It is a very popular food from southern India. Soak black gram dāl (without skins) and rice separately overnight. Use twice as much rice as dāl. The next day, take the rice and dāl out of the water and make a fine paste of them in a mixer. Mix well these two ingredients and leave the mixture overnight so it gets slightly fermented. You may add a little salt to it. To make *dosās*, spread a small quantity of this mixture in a hot pan that has a little oil in it.

Dosās should be very thin. They are made one at a time. To cook, turn them only once to cook the other side. *Dosās* may be eaten as they are, or they can be filled with various vegetables and rolled like crepes.

RICE

When rice is simply cooked in water, it is known as boiled rice. Measure the rice, wash and soak it in water for about 10 minutes. Then put it in boiling water which should be twice the quantity of the rice. To this water you may add seeds from two cardamoms, 2–3 cloves, and a piece of cinnamon for about $1\frac{1}{4}$ cups (250 grams) of rice, so that the rice does not imbalance the *vāta* and *kapha*. Cover it and let it cook on a low fire until all the water is evaporated. You may add some ghee or butter to the freshly prepared rice and keep it covered for a short while. This rice may be eaten with vegetables or with dāl. Alternatively, one may fry this rice with some vegetables in the following manner for a quick meal.

Vegetables and Rice

For a portion of rice for two persons, add 2 tablespoons of hot ghee, $\frac{1}{2}$ teaspoon of cumin seeds, 2 cloves, seeds from 2 cardamoms, 2 bay leaves, half a spoon of Spice Mixture A and an equal amount of salt. Add to this a chopped onion. Stir a little while frying. Add some finely cut vegetables to it. You may make the choice of vegetables according to your circumstances and requirements, but green peas, green beans, carrots, leeks, paprika, or mushrooms are good. Add also 2 teaspoons dried raisins. Keep stirring, and cook the vegetables without adding additional water. If some of the vegetables are slow to cook, leave them covered at a low fire. When the vegetables are cooked, add nearly as much the quantity of boiled rice as you have vegetables in the pot. Stir it all together until the rice is well mixed with the vegetables. Vegetable rice may be eaten with *rayāta* described on page 58.

Crushed Wheat with Vegetables

This is another recipe for a quick meal. Crushed wheat is available in health food stores. You may also make it yourself. For about $\frac{1}{2}$

cup (100 grams) of crushed wheat, fry an onion in ghee or oil and add to it ½ teaspoon each of salt, cumin seeds, and Spice Mixture A. You may add some green chili or red chili powder if you like it hot. Keep stirring and add some green peas, green beans, or other vegetables of your choice. When green vegetables are slightly cooked, add 2 chopped medium-sized tomatoes and 2 cloves garlic. After cooking a little, add the crushed wheat and stir well so that the wheat is mixed with vegetables. Add twice the quantity of water as wheat. Keep it covered and let all this cook over a low fire. Taste it to make sure that the wheat is well cooked. After it is cooked, keep it covered for a while before serving.

You may cook great millet or couscous with the same recipe.

DĀLS

Dāls are like soups, and are cooked in water with spices. When they are well cooked, they are seasoned with a preparation of ghee, onions, and more spices. Cleaned and washed dāls are added in the boiling water along with some salt, turmeric (curcuma), hot green chili, and fresh ginger. Some dāls, especially when they are full grain, take a very long time to cook, and water has to be added again and again. This time is shortened with the use of a pressure cooker. In any case, whatever dāl you may cook, make sure that it is well cooked and its grains are completely soft. Dāls without skin cook faster. Mung beans and masoor beans work best. I highly recommend the use of these two dāls because of their wholesome qualities. Urad beans take the longest to cook. Even in the pressure cooker, it takes 45 minutes to one hour. Black gram dāl is recommended as an aphrodisiac (see Part II).

Basic Dāl

For seasoning about ½ cup (100 grams) of dāl, add 3 tablespoons of ghee in a pot. When it is hot, add 1 spoon full of Spice Mixture B. After half a minute, add 2 medium-sized finely chopped onions and 1 tablespoon fresh ginger (if this was not added in the dāl earlier). When the onions are fried, add 3 to 4 cloves of garlic and 1 spoon of Spice Mixture A and some red chili powder if you like. When all this is fried, you may add 2 to 3 chopped tomatoes and cook them well. The addition of tomatoes is, however, optional; it is done to enhance the taste of the dāl. Add this seasoning to the dāl after it is cooked.

Masoor dāl (without skin) and mung dāl may be cooked with various vegetables. In some parts of India, it is a tradition to cook various dāls with vegetables, such as carrots, eggplants, beans, tomatoes, zucchini, etc. When all this is cooked, some spices are fried in ghee and added to it. It is very essential to add ghee and spices to the dāls, as otherwise dāls are hard to digest.

Dāl Soup

Dāl soup may be prepared with mung beans or masoor beans (without skin). For four persons, take ½ cup (100 grams) dāl, wash it, and add 5 cups boiling water. Chop 4 medium-sized carrots, 4 tomatoes, 2 onions and 4 cloves of garlic. Add the carrots and onions, ½ to 1 teaspoon salt, ½ teaspoon each anise, cumin, freshly crushed pepper, and coriander to the boiling dāl. When dāl and carrots are well-cooked, add the tomatoes and garlic, and cook for another 10 minutes. Add 3 tablespoons of butter or ghee after cooking.

PREPARING VEGETABLES AND EGGS

Some vegetables are prepared with sauce, whereas some others are just cooked with ghee or oil. You should eat a combination of vegetables rather than a single vegetable with your meals. For example, a combination of 2 carrots, 1 potato, a bit of cabbage, and a tomato is better than eating one of these vegetables each day. Mixed vegetables may be cooked with onions, ginger, a clove of garlic, and little bit of Spice Mixture A. Saute the onion and ginger first, then add the spices and salt and then the vegetables. Garlic should be added in the end.

You should always wash vegetables before cutting, and not the reverse. Always cut the vegetables into small pieces. This way, you save time and fuel because they cook faster and do not lose their taste and flavor. Besides, this method allows the spices to become better integrated in the vegetables, and they look more beautiful.

Try to learn to prepare food according to the seasons and your own basic constitution. For example, if it is too hot and you are cooking *pitta*-promoting vegetables, use more coriander and anise in your cooking. With practice, one learns to be more aware of various combinations and their subtle effect on the body. For preparing a wholesome diet, avoid extreme tastes in food. For example, do not eat foods that are extremely sour, sweet, salty, etc. Such extreme tastes alter the body's humors drastically and make one vulnerable to ailments.

Tomato Sauce

This basic sauce can be used for several vegetables. The quantities are for using a pound of tomatoes. This quantity of sauce is enough for a pound of green peas and the same weight of potatoes.

Take 4 medium-sized onions and cut them into small pieces, or crush them. Heat 3 tablespoons ghee or cooking oil in a pot and add to it 1 tablespoon finely cut or crushed ginger. After frying it a little, add the onions and keep cooking, stirring until you see that they are well-cooked and turning slightly brown. Add 1 teaspoon turmeric powder, 1½ teaspoons Spice Mixture A, 1 hot green chili (optional) and ½ to 1 teaspoon salt. The quantity of salt depends upon the vegetable you are going to cook, and upon your taste. Stir well and cook for a minute. Now add to it 6 tablespoons yogurt and keep stirring. Let it cook well for about five minutes and then add 1 pound of chopped tomatoes and 6 cloves of finely cut garlic. Cook them well until the sauce becomes well mixed.

Note: This sauce is delicious but a little heavy to digest. If you have weak digestive power, you should leave out the yogurt.

Green Peas and Potatoes

A popular vegetable prepared with tomato sauce is a combination of green peas and potatoes. For the above-described quantity of sauce, you can use about 1 pound green peas (without shells) and 2 to 3 medium-sized potatoes cut in small cubes. Cook these vegetables in the sauce for about half an hour. Chickpeas may also be prepared in this sauce. Cook them in water with a little salt until they are soft and then put them in the sauce. Cook the two together for at least half an hour and crush some chickpeas in the sauce. Potatoes alone may also be prepared in this sauce. Boil them with the skins and peel them afterward. Cut them into small pieces. Potatoes should be cooked with the above described sauce for about half an hour. In this preparation, the potatoes are nearly mashed in the sauce.

Baingan Bhartha (Eggplant)

Another nice preparation with this sauce includes eggplant. Take 2 pounds of nice round eggplants and cook them on all sides directly on the flame, or put them in the oven until they become soft. After that, peel off the skin and mash them well. Put this preparation into the tomato sauce, which should be made without yogurt. Mix well the sauce and the eggplant, and cook together for 15 minutes while constantly stirring. If you do not stir, it will stick to the surface, and if you do not cook long enough, it will not taste so good. This preparation is called *bainqan bhartha* in northwestern India.

There is another very simple and quick recipe for cooking certain vegetables. Cabbage or leafy vegetables, radishes, cauliflower, potatoes, turnips, or any combination of several of these may be cooked as follows. For about 1 pound of peeled vegetables, heat 2 tablespoons cooking oil in a pot and add to it 1 teaspoon of Spice Mixture B, $\frac{1}{2}$ teaspoon freshly ground coriander, and $\frac{1}{4}$ teaspoon red chili powder (optional). Add the vegetables quickly after the spices are cooked for a few seconds. Stir the vegetables and spices constantly. You may add salt according to taste and according to the nature of the vegetables. Even without salt, this preparation tastes very good.

Preparation of Eggs

Here is a simple preparation of eggs with some vegetables. For 4 eggs, cut 2 medium-sized onions and fry them in 3 tablespoons ghee. Add to it 2 teaspoons finely chopped ginger, $\frac{1}{2}$ teaspoon each of Spice Mixture A, freshly ground coriander seeds, and turmeric. Add also $\frac{1}{4}$ teaspoon salt, and cook everything together for a minute. Then add some green peas or some other vegetable. When the vegetables are cooked a little, add 2 medium-sized, finely chopped tomatoes. Cook all these for about 2–3 minutes and add whipped eggs in this preparation while stirring constantly. Cook for another minute.

Rāyatā

Rāyatā is a yogurt preparation which accompanies meals. According to Āyurvedic tradition, it should be eaten only during lunch and not for dinner. Different kinds of *rāyatās* are made by adding various things to whipped yogurt. You may add pieces of banana, boiled potatoes, tomatoes, grated cucumber, etc. Salt, pepper, and powdered cumin are added to this preparation to taste.

DESSERTS

According to Āyurvedic tradition, it is recommended to eat something sweet after meals. However, one should not eat desserts made from grains or other heavy ingredients after main meals. Desserts made of *chenā* (a cheese) and fruits are recommended. However, it does not mean that other desserts are not eaten. There are numerous preparations of sweets which are used for various purposes. Here are a few.

Germinating Wheat Starch

This dessert is strength-promoting and wholesome food. Wash and soak the wheat in water for about 24 hours. Crush it in a mixer and extract the starch by filtering it through a thin muslin cloth. To cook, add the starch to some ghee, and cook for about 15 minutes while stirring. Add twice the amount of milk as starch and 5 crushed cardamoms. Reduce the mixture to one third and add sugar (to taste), a few almonds, pistachio nuts, and raisins. This may be eaten cold in summer and hot in winter.

Khīr

Rice pudding is also popular now in the West, but it is made differently in India. Wash and soak ¾ cup (150 grams) rice for about 10 minutes. Put it in 2 cups boiling water and let it cook over a low fire. When most of the water has evaporated, add milk and 3–4 crushed cardamoms. Keep cooking for at least an hour on a slow fire and add more milk. You may use at least 4 cups or more of milk in the whole process. In the end, add some sugar according to taste, almonds, and pistachio nuts. *Khīr* may be eaten either cold or hot, depending upon the season.

Chenā Dessert

These desserts are prepared by cooking *chenā* in ghee while constantly stirring. In the section on milk products, I have already mentioned that *chenā* is made by adding lemon juice to boiling milk and then separating the milk solids. Cook *chenā* in ghee until it begins to get slightly brown. Add some sugar and finely powdered cardamom. You may add saffron instead of cardamom if you wish. Put the whole preparation on a plate and flatten it. Put finely cut almonds and pistachio nuts on the top. Let it cool and cut it into small pieces.

A variety of desserts are made from *chenā.* They are easier to digest than milk desserts or desserts prepared with various grain flours. Of particular importance are desserts made from Urad dal flour, which are aphrodisiacs. Some recipes are given in Part II.

ĀYURVEDIC DRINKS

Lassī

To make a sweet lassī, take a cup of yogurt and add 4 teaspoons of sugar (or according to taste). Add 3 cups of water and mix everything together with an egg-beater or a mixer. To make salty lassī, use 1 cup yogurt, $\frac{1}{2}$ teaspoon rock salt, $\frac{1}{4}$ teaspoon pepper, and 1 teaspoon of powdered cumin. Add 3 cups of water to your mixture and whip with an egg-beater or in your mixer. It is best to use cumin seeds for this. To make a powder, first roast them a little in a hot pan and then powder them in a hand grinder. Note: To roast something like this in a pan, just heat the pan and put the seeds in for a while. Do not use any oils when you do this. The seeds will "brown" a bit.

Spice Tea

Black tea is sour by nature, and too much tea vitiates *pitta*. The addition of various spices makes it a wholesome, strength-promoting and fatigue-alleviating drink. There are various combinations that can be added to the boiling water before the addition of the black tea. Following are the quantities of some ingredients for $1\frac{1}{4}$ cups (250 ml) water:

1. 2 crushed cardamoms;

2. 2 crushed cardamoms, 1 teaspoon grated or cut fresh ginger, and 2 crushed black peppers;

3. Half the seeds of one greater cardamom, a little piece of cinnamon, and 1 clove—all crushed together;

4. ¼ teaspoon anise.

Add any one of these mixtures to the water and when the water begins to boil, add

1½ teaspoons small-leaf black tea.

Let everything boil for half a minute.

Then add about ½ cup (100 ml) milk to it.

Add sugar according to taste and let everything boil together another half a minute.

Almond Milk

Almond milk may be prepared hot or cold. Soak 12 almonds in water for several hours. Peel them and crush them along with 2 cardamom seeds, a few grains of saffron, 3 pistachio nuts, and 2 teaspoons sugar (or according to taste). Make all this into a paste and stir it well in about 1½–2 cups (300 to 400 ml) of cold or hot milk.

Lemon Syrup

This is a preparation for making a wholesome cold or hot drink. Add 1 cup (1 kilo) sugar to 4 cups water along with ½ cup (100 grams) finely chopped ginger, 1 tablespoon anise seeds, and 14 crushed black pepper seeds. Cook all this together until it is turned into a thick syrup. It will take about half an hour. Keep stirring during the preparation. Cool it down and filter it. Add to it 14 powdered cardamoms and ¾ cup (150 ml) fresh lemon juice. Mix well and store in clean and dried bottles. Add a few spoons of this syrup to cold water in the summer, or to hot water in winter, as an appetizer or as a thirst reliever.

PART II

SEXUAL ENERGY AND ĀYURVEDIC TRADITION

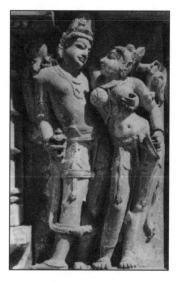

Vishnu-Lakshmi.

Lust was born first: neither gods, nor ancestors, nor humans can equal him. Oh Lust! you are immense as you reside in all living beings. I bow to you. . . . You are a higher deity than the sun, moon, wind and fire. . . . You are assimilated in all and therefore you are forever great. I bow to you.

Athārva Veda, IX, 2, 19, 24
1500 B.C.

4

INSTRUCTIONS FOR ENHANCING SEXUAL ENERGY

PERHAPS ONE CAN give sexuality the fourth important place after breathing, eating, and sleeping. Sleep is dealt with elsewhere[1] as this book intensifies our connection with the world of action. Sleep is a pause which temporarily disconnects us from worldly activities.

It has been already stated that the three humors are responsible for the physical and mental functions of the body. The resultant materials of these three humors are termed *dhātus*. There are seven *dhātus* and *śukra dhātu* is responsible for sexual activities, sexual excretions, procreation, and all the allied functions. This *dhātu* is described in a recent Āyurvedic book in Sanskrit:

> *Śukradhātu* is not expressed during childhood and dries up in old age. Like a full bloom, it is in blossom and sensuous during youth. It is produced in monthly cycles. Its chief function is to provide sensuous pleasure, fondness, and pregnancy.[2]

It has been said earlier that holistically everything is interconnected and interrelated. For a healthy body and healthy mind it is absolutely essential to have humoral balance, and the proper functioning of all the *dhātus*. One disorder or malfunction leads to another, and if proper care is not taken, one gets into a vicious cycle of health problems. According to Āyurveda, the non-fulfillment of desires, and facing the undesired, are two causes of psy-

---

[1] I have cited my basic book on Āyurveda for details of some concepts which are not a part of this book. Please see *Ayurveda: A Way of Life* (York Beach, ME: Samuel Weiser, 1995).

[2] P. V. Sharma, *Ṣoḍaśaṅgahṛdayam*, in Sanskrit and Hindi (Varanasi: Padmā Prakaśan, 1989), p. 13.

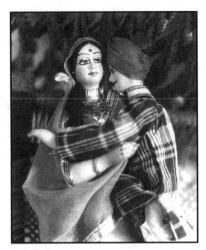

Figure 7. A doll couple from Bihar, northern India.

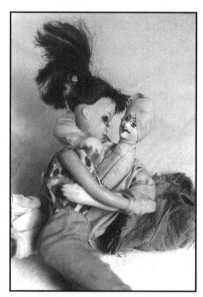

Figure 8. Amorous dolls. Cross-cultural German doll with an Indian man from Maharashtra.

chic problems.[3] However, this should not be misunderstood, as I do not mean to convey that one should be devoid of restraint and self-control. On the contrary, the Āyurvedic tradition lays a great emphasis on exercising control over one's senses.

Sexuality can be compared to food and nutrition in many respects. In nutrition, excess and a lack of certain components causes imbalance and ill health. Eating too little causes serious malnutrition problems and diseases, whereas eating too much gives rise to another set of diseases. A balance is absolutely essential. The same is true for sexual indulgence.

With the right ingredients, and with a little effort, one can prepare a variety of delicious foods to delight one's palate. On the other hand, with negligence and a lack of involvement, one can prepare insipid and uninspiring food with the same ingredients. Eating a delicious meal will lead to a sense of fulfillment and pleasure. Balanced and well-prepared food will provide vitality and vigor, whereas insipid or imbalanced food will give rise to dissatisfaction and indigestion. Think how this applies to sexuality!

When we eat quickly, we are gulping down our food in a state of stress that will create more stress and cause discomfort. When the same food is properly chewed and eaten peacefully, it provides energy. The same concept applies to sexual behavior: performance is very important here, too. In both cases, what plays the most important role is what we call, in Sanskrit, *bhāvanā*. *Bhāvanā* is a mixture of intention and feeling. Whether it is the preparation of food or a sexual relationship, the addition of *bhāvanā* brings life to all.

Food regenerates and revitalizes the body, whereas sexuality procreates. Eating food is a social activity and is associated with sharing. Sexuality also involves complete sharing and intimacy. But sexuality leads to a moment of great intensity. It evokes inner dormant energy. It takes us from the outer (phenomenal world) to the inner (eternal, indestructible self) momentarily. With training of the mind, one can learn to prolong this momentary stillness, and experience a link with cosmic immensity. Our eternal energy is the cause of our being. By transcending the phenomenal world, and connecting ourselves with the cosmic immensity, we expand our power, or *śakti*, and develop extrasensory perception.

---

[3] *Caraka Saṃhitā, Sūtrasthāna,* XI, 45.

The sexual experience begins with physical fondness, closeness, and sharing. However, through the physical, it transcends the physical, leading to a moment of bliss. This bliss, or *ananda*, gives us an experience of the eternal. With a determination to achieve this goal, by breaking away from mechanized notions that pervade all aspects of our living, and by adopting an attitude of sanctity toward the union of the opposites, one can convert the sexual experience into a blissful cosmic experience of eternity. You will realize that sexuality means much more than momentary sensuous pleasure, constricted and constrained by various social impositions. The soul is free by nature, and so is the cosmos. With all the possible scientific and technological developments of our age, we are still not able to manipulate natural forces. We cannot order time to stop, the Earth to move slower or faster, or the sun to rise when we want it to. We must realize all this and rejoice in our eternal freedom and accept the bliss of nature.

Lest I be misunderstood, I want to make it clear that I am not referring to the much talked about "sexual freedom" in the West. This has a very superficial aspect and has caused tremendous social problems. What I mean here by freedom is our inherent liberty to express our entire being, to let it be free with the cosmic rhythm, to join the eternal cosmic dance. This can only be achieved by getting rid of our self-imposed constraints. We suppress the inner light within us with an envelope of darkness, which is our own ignorance. It is up to us to develop an ability to see this inner light and to live an enlightened life. Our ability or power to think and decide *(buddhi)* is our freedom. We can use this freedom to harmonize our existence with the nature of the soul which is totally free and eternal.

I know that in our age of fast food, supersonic ways of traveling, and satellite communication systems, the reader is getting impatient with this philosophical discussion, and wants to quickly know about ready-made Āyurvedic formulas for obtaining more "sexual joy." But you must know that in holistic medicine, which is, in fact, a holistic way of being, there is no quick pill to immediately remove the symptoms of our troubles. According to the holistic way, removing symptoms is not a cure. In the holistic system, nature is a pharmaceutical company and the fastest pill here is to learn a simple formula; that is, to harmonize oneself with the natural order of things. This discussion is intended to make you pause a little bit, to make you aware of yourself and to achieve a moment of stillness. It is this moment of stillness which you can learn to prolong through sexuality.

SEXUAL BALANCE IN THE CONTEXT OF ĀYURVEDA

Three humors which govern all the physical and mental functions of the body are responsible for different aspects of sexual expression, and the humoral equilibrium is essential for sexual fulfillment and healthy children.

As you know, *vāta* is mobile, and is responsible for all body movement. In the context of sexuality, *vāta* is responsible for the sex act and sexual retention. If *vāta* is vitiated, both the sexual act and retention are affected adversely. One feels fatigued and breathless rather quickly, and the power of retention is considerably diminished.

Pitta is responsible for sexual vigor. An imbalance of *pitta* leads to a lack of initiative for sexual activity. It gives rise to all those problems that make one sexually less desirable. It may give rise to body odors, tearing and thickening of the skin, rashes, acne, herpes, etc.

Kapha is responsible for sexual potency. Vitiation of this humor leads to diminished or abnormal sexual excretions. This may give rise to abnormal progeny or sterility. In the technologically advanced and highly industrialized nations, the dominating humor is *vāta*.[4] When there is too much *vāta*, it dries up *kapha*, which results in the lack of sexual excretions. This latter gives rise to multiple sexual problems. It hinders the most important phenomenon of nature—procreation. In highly industrialized nations, 10 percent of the couples are incapable of having children. After Europe and America, this percentage is rapidly catching up in Japan. Besides this, couples suffer from problems due to a lack of sexual excretions, thereby giving rise to other social problems. I will treat this subject again later on.

---

[4] See *Ayurveda: A Way of Life.*

For a healthy sexual life, one needs balance. What follows are guidelines and tonics that are known to enhance sexual attraction and energy.

Regular inner and outer cleaning is absolutely essential for complete sexual expression. A person with constipation, a bad stomach, or an accumulation of similar ailments will have varied sexual problems. Most people are not aware of these simple facts, and they suffer in silence. Another thing to be aware of relates to the evacuative therapy described in my first book. Excessive evacuation may cause weakness, and a lack of sexual vigor and desire. Other instructions will be given later. Right now, I will treat certain specific aspects in relation to sexual attraction and energy.

BEAUTY

In Āyurveda, it is said that there is no greater aphrodisiac than a beautiful person.[5] Beauty in the present context does not mean abiding to some set concept in a particular society that describes particular features, complexion, etc. Beauty is meant in a wider medical sense. It is the radiance of a person; it is a smooth and healthy skin, clean body parts, pleasant smells, brightness in the eyes, clean nails, well dressed hair, and other such features. To take a concrete example, a person suffering from constipation (a *vāta* ailment) cannot really look beautiful, as he or she will have rough skin and a dull complexion. Similarly, vitiated *vāta* may give rise to a hoarse voice, yawning, and hiccups. All these features take away the beauty of a person.

A person with a vitiated *pitta* may suffer from bad skin, acne, herpes, etc., and does not look attractive and beautiful. He or she may also have bad breath, and body odor. This makes a person sexually unattractive in the context of the subject we are discussing. The vitiation of *kapha* makes one dull and lazy rather than active and beautiful. One has a lack of initiation and some-

---

[5] In Āyurvedic literature, there is a mention of a beautiful woman being the best aphrodisiac. This view is understandable because this literature was compiled by men, and they wrote from their frame of reference. I have especially paid attention to this, and have considered both the man's and woman's context.

times suffers from depression. The body movements are not elegant and swift.

In brief, beauty in the present context means that one has smooth skin, which is not too oily and not too dry, a bright complexion, expressive eyes, clean body parts, a pleasant smell from the body and an agreeable voice. Well kept and well dressed hair are equally essential for an attractive and desirable look.

I will describe below some of the measures you should undertake to acquire an attractive and appealing look. I wish to make two important points before proceeding further. 1) The measures to maintain external beauty described below are in addition to keeping the humors in equilibrium. One also needs to regularly clean the body externally and internally. You cannot look either sexually attractive or enjoy fully the sexual act if your intestines are filled with accumulated excreta, your breath smells because of liver problems, stomach disorders, or other similar features. 2) Nearly all over the world, and particularly in Western countries, measures of beauty are described only for women. This is also evident from the media. It is essential for the readers to remove this discrimination from their minds. A yawning, tired looking man, with rough skin and hair, with dull eyes is as unattractive for a woman as the woman with the similar features for a man. It is a different story if a woman, due to cultural and social suppression, does not express herself and accepts the undesirable. Āyurvedic instructions on sexual behavior are for an expansion of sexual energy. This is only possible when both partners are completely uninhibited and free in expressing themselves. Fondness begins at the physical level, and if there is any hindrance at this stage, it inhibits sexual expression in one way or the other. Men should not ignore this section on beauty and should know that women also like men to be attractive.

ENHANCING SENSUOUS POWER

One also gets stimulated like a bull by massage, anointing, baths, perfumes, garlands, adorations, a comfortable house, bed and chairs, good, attractive clothes, the chirping of happy birds, the tinkling of ornaments on women, and the gentle pressing of the body.[6]

---

[6] *Caraka Saṃhitā, Cikitsāsthānam*, II (3), 24–25.

Sexuality begins with sensuality. During the sexual process, one slowly transcends the senses. In other words, all five senses are used, and it is their coordination that accounts for the intensity of sexual pleasure. For enhancing sexual pleasure, or expanding one's sexual energy or power *(kāmaśakti)*, the first step is to augment the power of individual senses with various practices. We will discuss these individually.

Touch

The tactile sensation of the body, the sense of touch, plays an important role in sexuality. It is not only physiological tactile sensation, but the energy radiations around the body which emerge from the *hṛdya* (see next section for details of *hṛdya*). Thus, there is also something on the surface of our skin. One must make sure that all the fine energy channels located at the surface of the skin are open. The skin is very sensitive to *vāta* vitiation, which makes it rough by blocking these energy channels. That means that blocked energy channels do not let the nourishment reach the surface.

To take appropriate care of the skin, first of all, you must clean it properly. You must not always clean yourself with soap as soap dries the skin and enhances *vāta*. Rub your body with full cream milk two or three times a week to nourish your skin. Milk cleans very well and replaces soap. Preferably, the milk should be fresh cows' milk, and not homogenized or processed. Take milk in an open utensil, and with your hand, apply it and rub it on each part of your body. If you feel that some parts of your body have excessively rough skin, apply full cream yogurt with active bacteria. Yogurt also cures minor infections and makes the skin slightly oily. If you cannot buy fresh milk from a farm, commercial milk can be used. You can find natural yogurt in health food stores.

Your nails should be cut regularly, and you should take special care of your hands and feet. They should be regularly and properly oiled. Armpits should be well cleaned. The hair should be removed from time to time. The sex organs should be well cleaned and washed with a warm water shower. Women should wash the vagina with some kind of hand douche or enema apparatus.[7]

---

[7] See *Ayurveda: A Way of Life.*

For enhancing tactile sensations, it is important to have a regular oil massage. It is not necessary to go to a masseuse for it. You can exchange a massage with family or friends, or oil your body yourself. It is highly recommended to saturate your body with oil once a week. Use an Āyurvedic massage oil with a sesame base, or hot ghee, almond oil, or coconut oil. Rub the oil on each part of your body systematically. Rub hard so that the skin can absorb it. Once you have finished oiling the whole body, look at the part from where you started. You will realize that the skin has already absorbed a considerable amount. Repeat the process. Like this, oil your body two to four times by rubbing strongly each time. After you finish, it is recommended to wipe off the extra oil with a hot wet hand towel. Do not take a shower immediately. This treatment makes the skin soft like a baby's, enhances sensitivity, and gives strength against injuries and shock. *This treatment is not recommended for people who are excessively overweight or who suffer from depression or other* kapha *ailments.*

While massaging and cleaning, you should pay special attention to hands and feet. Some people tend to be negligent about their feet. In the cold countries, it is thought that the feet are covered anyway, why beautify them? However, in the present context, you must take care of your feet and enhance their tactile sensation. Feet can be used as much as hands in sexual activity, and should be massaged regularly to enhance their sensitivity.

Besides the care of the skin, a regular body massage makes you aware and sensitive to your physical self. This is essential for complete sexual expression. You must always keep in mind that sexuality is not limited to certain parts of the body. For the expansion of sexual energy, every part of your body should participate in enhancing and channeling the sexual energy.

Sight

Sharpening the sense of sight is to develop keen observation. For complete self-expression, you must develop a sharp sense of observation and the capacity to observe the reactions of your actions on your partner and then act in an appropriate way. All this is done by observing the gestures, expressions, and sensations of the other person. By sharpening one's sensitivity in this direc-

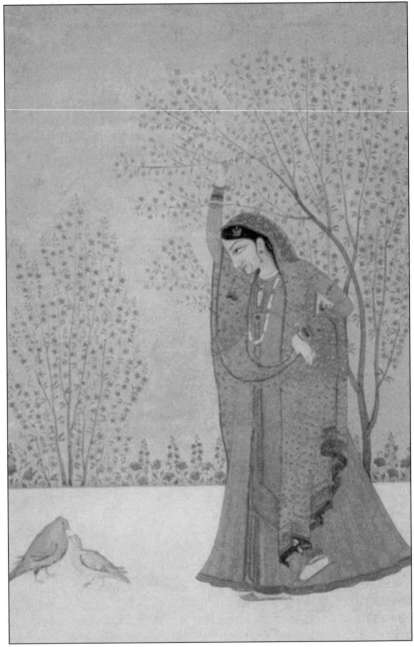

Figure 9. Engrossed in thoughts of her lover, the lady is watching two amorous pigeons. Kangara School. Rekha Jhanji Collection.

tion, one spontaneously observes the most minute details of one's actions and the reactions of the other. However, one should not be tense or overly careful about observing the other. This will have a contrary effect and will give rise to other complications.

Let us see how you can learn to develop a sharp sense of observation. This process should not begin with your partner, as this means that you are beginning with a limitation. When I talk of sharpening your senses, it cannot be done in limited circumstances. It applies to life in general. You cannot just learn to observe the changing expressions of some people and not notice that a house around the corner on your street has been demolished. You must learn to keenly observe all things around you. You must begin to observe trees, birds, sky and its changing colors; you must observe the increasing and decreasing moon and other natural phenomena. You must learn to observe people around you very carefully—their expressions, the fatigue on their faces, changes in weight, complexion, etc. You must go through life with "open eyes." This is only possible by learning to live in the present moment. This is the key to enhance sensitivity as well as *kāmaśakti* (sexual energy). Learn to fully concentrate on whatever you are doing. It may be a mundane activity, like cleaning your teeth, taking a shower, or talking to others. Be interested in your surroundings and the people around you. Listen to them carefully when they talk. Observe the animals in your surroundings; observe the little seedlings grow, observe the seasonal changes in the trees around you; learn to observe *all*. Live life in its intensity. Do not go through life with your eyes closed.

An enhanced sense of observation is essential at every step of sexual communication. If you did not notice the new dress or the missing beard, and your partner was looking forward to your comments, it already speaks for a bad beginning. If you are to learn to enhance your sexual energy, begin by seeing.

Smell, Taste, and Hearing

You need to sharpen the power of your senses if you are to enhance sexual energy. The three senses play an important role.

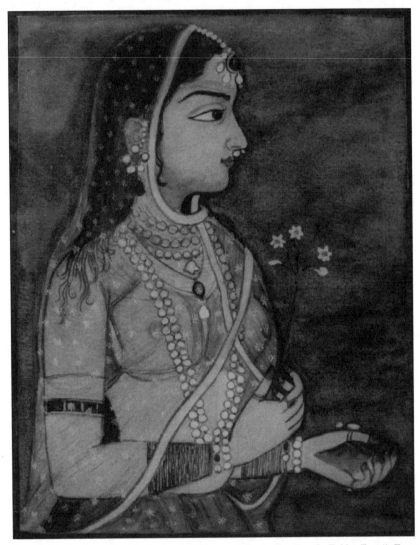

Figure 10. Lady waiting for her lover. Kangara School. Painting by Rekha Jhanji. From author's collection.

Smell is important for many reasons. If your body smells bad, people don't want to be near you. Body odor is an anaphrodisiac (a word that expresses what is contrary to an aphrodisiac). In Āyurvedic literature, many products are mentioned because they smell good, and have an aphrodisiac effect. The body smell of certain persons is highly pleasant and sexually exciting, whereas others are repelling. Your body odor depends upon your humoral constitution, and it is possible to change it. The body smell can be changed and made pleasant and sexually exciting by keeping the humors balanced. You have to learn to eat the appropriate combinations of nutrients.

The sense of smell can be enhanced by developing your sensitivity. Everything has an odor. Make it a habit to see and feel the things around you, and to recognize them from their smells. Blind people have a very enhanced sense of smell and touch, which helps to overcome the loss of sight. However, the enhanced sense of smell also has a negative side. A bad smell from your partner may put you off very quickly. But, as I said before, the body smell can be altered and made pleasant and appealing.

We are all aware that it is the pleasant and aphrodisiac effect of certain substances on which the whole perfume industry is based. There are unaccountable varieties of smells in our universe, and unlike visual objects and speech, we have no recording system for them. Rose, jasmine, water lily, sandalwood, etc., are exhilarating smells. However, the variation in nature is tremendous. Pleasant and subtle smells of the flowers of linden, albizzia, and citrus are less universally known, but are extremely sensuous and desire-provoking.

There are also distinguishable smells from various places: smell the earth when water falls on it, be by the sea shore and smell the salt air. There are flavors from innumerable food products all over the world, such as the smell of coffee, or garlic, or the smell of good chai (tea). For these latter, the two senses participate simultaneously—the sense of smell and taste.

People who are keen observers have sharp and developed minds. They enjoy each aspect of life. As I have discussed earlier, an individual is an integrated whole, part of this dynamic, ever-changing universe, and cannot live a fragmented existence. A person who cannot sit and enjoy a good meal is usually not sensuous

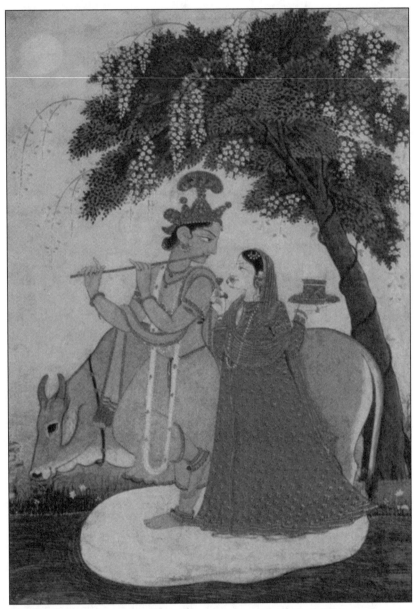

Figure 11. Krishna and Radha. Kangara School. Rekha Jhanji's Collection.

in other aspects of life. To evoke fully the sexual energy, one simultaneously uses all the senses.

To enhance the sense of taste, begin to recognize a variety of food from its flavor and taste. Things foreign to you, like exotic spices or fruits, may be tasted in small quantities. Keep them in your mouth and close your eyes. Slowly try to concentrate on the experience and sensation they provide you. Do not try to compare them with a taste and smell you already know. Just try to have the sensation first. The names can be learned later on.

Hearing can be enhanced like the rest of the senses. A fine sensitivity to sound, learning to discriminate between various nuances of words, melodies, and the natural sounds of this universe lead you to attain enhanced auditory capabilities. This happens when you speak several languages, or have learned music, or develop a kind of hypersensitivity to sound due to the heightened awakening of auditory perception.

In the living tradition of India, other sounds than music play an important role in enhancing sexual energy. Sound is considered very powerful, fragile, and delicate. It is associated with *śakti* (power or strength) which is the eternal female energy. Fine sounds are associated with women and reveal their presence and actions, their gestures and movements. Therefore, jewelry for women is designed to look and sound beautiful. A man's imagery of a woman, whether it is his mother, sister, or wife, is associated with subtle sounds of bangles, anklets, earrings, and other jewelry worn by her. From the variations of the sounds due to gestures, he is able to recognize which woman member of his family is there. This may sound strange to the readers in the West, as all this is foreign to their culture. It reminds me of comments from my several European friends saying that a sari must be an uncomfortable dress because one has to adjust again and again its free hanging part on the shoulder. In fact, for Indian men, these are romantic gestures that are associated with the sound of a woman's bangles when she adjusts her sari.

In addition to the sounds of women's jewelry, there are sounds of birds, music, adoration, soft sweet words, etc., which enhance the sexual energy in both men and women. Make an effort to develop sensitivity to sound. Listen to non-specific sounds very carefully. Try to distinguish them from each other. Try to recognize people from their footsteps. Try to recognize things and actions from their sounds only. Listen to the singing of various birds and learn to distinguish them. We all know that training in music enhances sensitivity to sound.

I have talked about evoking the power of one's senses so you develop a high level of sensitivity and can use them in evoking sexual energy to the maximum. However, I do want to warn you that the developed senses can be a nuisance in our technologically advanced age where there are so many harsh sounds, unpleasant smells, and distorted tastes. On the other hand, if you keep your sensitivity dull for fear of unpleasantness, then you can never achieve the most profound sexuality and learn to transcend sensuality through sensuality. An additional positive aspect from evoking the strength of the senses *(indrivaśakti)* is that you may also grow sensitive to environmental catastrophes and collectively try to save our planet from destruction.

ENHANCING SEXUAL CAPABILITY

Sexual energy is considered very powerful and it is advised not to suppress it. However, it is possible to channel it with conscious effort. Suppression or lack of an appropriate expression of sexual energy may give rise to several physical and/or mental ailments.

> A conscious person should use aphrodisiacs regularly because virtue, wealth, pleasure, and fame depend on them.[8]

Āyurvedic texts explain various categories of substances that act to enhance sexual vigor, fertility, the sexual impulse, retention, and sexual excretions. Since this book is meant for the general reader, I will not go into the technical details. It is important to define what is meant by an aphrodisiac in Āyurvedic terms. An aphrodisiac is that substance, action, or factor which enhances one or more of the following: sexual vigor, fertility, sexual impulse, retention, sexual excretions, and sexual attraction. On the contrary, an anaphrodisiac (a coined word) is a substance, ac-

---

[8] *Caraka Saṃhitā, Cikitsāsthānam,* II, (3), 24–25.

tion, or factor that will diminish one or more of the above de-scribed attributes.

Our principal concern is to learn about aphrodisiacs in order to use them to enhance the sexual energy. However, the knowl-edge of anaphrodisiacs is also important for two reasons: 1) to avoid factors with an anaphrodisiac effect so they do not become a hindrance in sexual expression; 2) sometimes there is a big dif-ference between the sex drive of two partners, and the excessive sexual vigor of one partner becomes a hindrance for sexual com-patibility. In such cases, to reach a suitable level with each other, the use of anaphrodisiac products will be required.

In fact, all substances that function as anaphrodisiacs will be discussed so you can avoid them.

Anaphrodisiac Factors and Substances

Our modern mechanized way of living is one of the greatest anaphrodisiacs. In highly industrialized and technologically ad-vanced nations, and in big cities of the world, people are timed like machines. They experience overwork, stress, tension, and ex-cessive running around. Everything is pre-planned and well-defined. There is no spontaneity in life. There is no time to observe the trees and the flowers, or to listen to the birds, or the sounds of water and wind, or enjoy the moon or the rising and setting sun. In fact, many city dwellers do not even know about the phases of the moon. They work in closed places with artificial light and climatic conditions. There is well-defined leisure time but that, too, is generally filled with activities. There is no real leisure when people are free of anxiety and the notion of "doing something." In these circumstances, sexuality has lost its real sanctity and is also considered as one of the activities which can fit in a routine. It is no longer a natural and spontaneous sharing between two persons. Like the Saturday shopping, it is more or less a fixed routine. Since people are not relaxed and their lives are hectic, they are unable to concentrate, lack innovation and imagination, and think that sexual activity is like a mechanical ac-tivity which should be able to work well on command. They have a mechanical "switch on and switch off" attitude. Somehow, the natural phenomena do not work like that. Just as we cannot

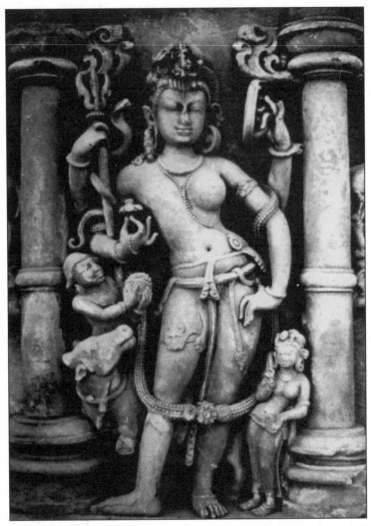

Figure 12. Ardhanariśvra from Khajuraho. It is the symbol of male-female union.

order the sun to rise in the middle of the night and have spring during winter, similarly, sexual desire and impulse have appropriate conditions and time.

Due to the environmental pollution, there are holes in the protective ozone layer of the atmosphere and because of that the sun's rays can cause skin cancer. Similarly, with a mechanized way of living, we have made sacred sexual activity, which is the base of propagating human life on this Earth, full of problems. When sexual energy is blocked, it also blocks the other energy channels in the body. There is a lack of sexual excretion, desire but no impulse, sexual vigor diminishes, and the retention period is short. When these problems persist over a long time, they may give rise to serious physiological or mental diseases. Thus, you should not think the problems of sexuality are only limited to sexual pleasure.

An Āyurvedic way of life makes us aware of our being and leads to self-realization. Sexuality involves two people and a oneness of their complementary energies takes place during the sex act. There is a strong flow of energy between two beings who make love. You must transcend yourself completely during the sexual act and need to get over any restrictions and restraints. Otherwise, it is not possible to reach the state of oneness, or to have the experience of being one with the cosmic energy.

In our times, another factor that acts as an anaphrodisiac is the spread of pornography and the commercialization of, and disrespect for, a woman's body. It may sound ironic, for pornography is meant to be an aphrodisiac. Seeing pictures of naked women or sex-oriented scenes in the media, or the display of other sex-related images, causes a slow release of sexual energy, which ultimately causes a lack of vigor. Subtlety, mystique, and respect have vanished. People have acquired a "consumer's" attitude toward sex. There is an emphasis on quantity rather than quality. Attention, patience, love, care, and respect, which are essential for sexual fulfillment, have diminished in people's minds. I feel that in this respect, we all (including modern day Indians) have a lot to learn from the ancient Indians who gave an equally holy place to eroticism and spirituality. The erotic sculptures were built on the temples, emphasizing the sensuous aspect of our existence. It was considered essential to recognize, accept, and go through the sensuous reality in order to attain ultimate spiritual liberation. It was

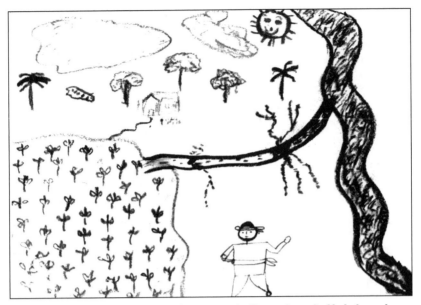

Figure 13. Obstacles that block sexual energy are similiar to those of a blocked canal.

not recommended to suppress sensuous reality and sexuality, but to experience it.

The yogis or ascetics who left worldly activities to attain spiritual liberation, and who went to the caves in the Himalayas, had to work very hard on themselves through various yogic practices to win over their senses completely. This was considered the hardest thing to do and the greatest to achieve as a human being. There are also stories about when the ascetics did not succeed in channeling their sexual energy, and had to return to the sensuous phenomenal world to attain the experience of senses in order to win over them. The erotic sculptures on the temples depict several stories to illustrate these profound philosophical ideas. Like this, the sanctity of the man-woman relationship was kept, and it was a highly respected binding. There were many ceremonies to make the sexual act a conscious and spiritual act.

Another factor harmful to sexuality is the slow social change from extended families to nuclear families, and the lack of customs and rituals. Perhaps it is not possible to follow the ancient rituals exactly, but we can modify them. Rituals lead to self-awareness and realization, they give us a consciousness of life which is essential in the present context.

In a single family unit, a couple may spend too much time together. This may cause social and sexual imbalance. Different aspects of sharing—sharing with mother, father, or other people—are all concentrated on one person, and the partner becomes the target for all kinds of emotional outlets. This weighs heavy on the sexual sharing of the two persons. In addition, the complete freedom of being alone makes some couples overindulgent; they lose the sanctity of this relationship and acquire a consumers' attitude toward this sacred aspect of life. I suggest that people make a conscious effort not to be alone all the time. They can invite parents, relatives, or friends to live with them. You will see that this will work like a rejuvenating therapy for your relationship. When two people are always together, they have too much of each other, and they begin to criticize and condemn each other. With the presence of other people in the family, they learn patience, begin to see the positive points of each other, and learn to appreciate each other more. Due to a limitation of private time, there is an accumulation of sexual energy which helps in opening the blocked channels, and this leads to a higher level of sexual communication than just a routine sex experience.

Another hindrance in sexuality and self-expression in this direction is caused by childbirth. The arrival of a baby makes a big change in the life of a couple. However, it should not damage the sexual communication of the parents. It happens because the woman, as a mother, acquires a greater role than the wife she was, and she becomes overindulgent to her baby, ignoring other aspects of her life. This is very damaging for her in the long run, as it has serious consequences in the later years of her life. She should not try to merge her identity with the baby. It is true that a baby is an integral part of the mother for nine months, but after childbirth, she should realize that her relationship with the baby should be like other relationships. It should not engulf her identity and consume all her time. She must learn to organize herself. She should not shower all her affection and energy on the baby and make grounds for future problems in her life. She must learn to let the baby out of her mind from time to time, and enjoy the bliss of sexuality with her partner.

On the part of the man, he should be understanding of the arrival of a third person in the family, should share the work of caring for the baby, building a relationship with the baby, and making an effort to revitalize every aspect of sharing with his partner. The couple could use some aphrodisiacs during this period. It is particularly necessary for the woman, who undergoes physiological and psychological changes with the childbirth.[9]

Another factor which acts as an anaphrodisiac is the intake of sedatives or sleeping pills. In our modern times, many people are unable to sleep. Sedatives generally have an anaphrodisiac effect. Their effect on sexuality is not due to the fact that they lull you to sleep. They have a very slow acting effect on your whole body, which gradually causes a lack of desire, impulse, retention, and sexual secretions. Therefore, if you have problems sleeping, take recourse to other measures described earlier rather than swallowing a pill.

These are just some of the factors that act as anaphrodisiacs and cause hindrances in sexual energy. We must make every effort to remove these obstacles. Without removing these, it is not wise to take aphrodisiac preparations. Imagine that you are paving a canal to direct water from the source to your fields. Before paying attention to the level of the paved canal for a free flow of water, you will make sure that there are no obstructions, such as stones or sand in the canal. Making an appropriate canal surface for a free flow of water would be the second step. Even if the level of your canal is well-manned and capable of bringing water to your fields, if there are big stones in the canal, all your efforts to make the surface level will be useless. The water will not reach its destination due to the obstructions, and your effort to make a canal will be futile.

There are several anaphrodisiac products that may be required to calm down the sexual impulse and vigor in certain cases. The simplest and most easily available is coriander. You need to take 1 teaspoon of powdered coriander seeds daily for a few days. If you are unable to eat the powder, make a decoction by adding 1 teaspoon of coriander in 1 cup (200 ml) water and reducing it to $\frac{1}{4}$ cup by cooking over a low fire. Do not buy already powdered or old coriander. Crush the seeds shortly before

---

[9] V. Verma, *Kāmasūtra for Women* (Munich: Scherz Verlag, 1994).

use. Do not think that eating coriander in a mixture of spices will give you this effect, as most of the other spices in those mixtures you have learned about in the previous section have aphrodisiac qualities.

Generally, herbal drugs with a bitter taste will have an anaphrodisiac effect. It is observed that people with excessive sexual desire tend to eat an aphrodisiac diet, such as ginger, garlic, spicy foods, or old sweet wine, sweet foods and drinks. Cutting the aphrodisiac foods will also help decrease the excessive sexual impulse and vigor.

APHRODISIAC MEASURES

Most of the Āyurvedic literature was written by *ṛṣis* (male sages). It is not that women did not play a role in medicine and health care paractices in India. Quite the contrary, in the family traditions and rituals even now, it is usually a wise woman of the family who knows all sorts of different formulations for health care, massage, yogic therapies, and preventive and curative nutrition. In fact, Āyurveda survives in Indian homes today because of the greatness of our women for keeping this tradition alive. But what I wish to mention in the present context is that the ancient literature on the subject of aphrodisiacs was written by men from their viewpoint, and this is also true about the treatises on sex, such as the *Kāmasūtra* and *Anaṇgaraṇga*. The following quotation is very amusing and informative in this direction.

> Due to the great diversity in people and the fortune of women, the feminine qualities, like a good appearance, are enhanced on finding a suitable man. The woman who is excellent in terms of age, beauty, voice, and amorous movements enters into the heart quickly and is like celebration of the heart. A woman who has a similar mind and psyche to her male partner is submissive, pleased with what he likes, and is like a noose for all the senses due to her excellent qualities. Separated from this woman, the man feels restlessly that the world is devoid of women, without her his body seems vacant of senses, finding her he is no more subdued with grief, agitation, restlessness, or fear; finding her he feels solace and seeing her, he is exhilarated, and meets her sexually ever as fresh due to his strong sexual urges, and even when he has frequent intercourse he does not get contented.

This is the best aphrodisiac for a man. Men differ in their psychological behavior. The healthy man who desires progeny should go to a
woman who belongs to dissimilar clan, who is stimulating, exhilarating, free from complications, and clean.[10]

It is interesting to know that the Āyurvedic sages learned a lot
from nature and they observed carefully the behavior of animals.
In fact, many medicines derived from plants were developed after
observing that the animals used to cure themselves with them.
Similarly, for sexual behavior, animal postures were copied and
some animal food was used to enhance sexual activity and retention. Of particular importance are the horse, bull, and elephant.
In fact, for the lack of sexual desire, it is advised to observe these
animals or to hang their pictures in the sleeping chamber.

In Āyurveda, there are many recipes to make aphrodisiacs. If
you are unable to get all the ingredients of a certain formulation,
do not feel discouraged. Take whatever is available. In any case,
these mixtures are very effective, as you will realize from some of
the citations given later.

I mentioned earlier that Āyurvedic literature is addressed to
men, but most of these aphrodisiacs are effective for both men
and women.

Aphrodisiacs should be used only after purifying the body
and cleaning the internal channels. Otherwise, they will not be effective. I have described the external cleaning and internal purification practices elsewhere. It is said in Āyurveda that, "At first, one
should apply evacuative therapy according to one's strength.
Aphrodisiacs do not succeed if taken in a dirty body just like a
dirty cloth does not take the dye properly."[11]

APHRODISIAC RECIPES

Enhance Sexual Energy

Boil *śāli* rice, add some ghee and salt. Eat this with black gram
soup (see section on nutrition). After eating this, take a glass of

---

[10] *Caraka Saṃhitā, Cikitsāsthānam*, II, (1), 8–15.
[11] *Caraka Saṃhitā, Cikitsāsthānam*, II, (1), 50–51.

hot, sweetened milk. The one who eats this "remains awakened with sexual impulse the whole night."[12] Note: Śāli rice may be difficult to find. If this is the case, use a short grain white rice (not Basmati rice).

Rejuvenating Sexual Engergy

Śāli rice ($\frac{1}{4}$ cup or 50 grams) should be sprinkled with $\frac{1}{4}$ cup (50 ml) milk and mashed in a mortar by constantly adding more milk so that the preparation remains moist and a fine paste is made. Afterward, add $\frac{3}{4}$ cup (150 ml) milk, stir and extract the juice from this preparation. Cook this juice in $\frac{1}{2}$ cup (100 ml) milk again. Separately, fry 2 tablespoons black gram flour in 1 tablespoon ghee and add the above preparation to it along with 2 tablespoons sugar. Stir on a low fire until it is semisolid. Then add 1 tablespoon each minced almonds, raisins, and dates, along with $\frac{1}{2}$ teaspoon powdered ginger, and $\frac{1}{4}$ teaspoon ground pepper. Stir the whole preparation over a low fire for 2–3 minutes. When it is cold, add 4 tablespoons honey to it. This can be preserved for a few days at low temperature. One should take 2 soupspoons of it with hot milk every day. It is strength-promoting, rejuvenating, and an aphrodisiac.

A Practical Aphrodisiac

A very simple and practical preparation is made by frying Urad dāl flour in one third its quantity of śāli rice flour in ghee. Take 3 tablespoons Urad dāl flour and 1 tablespoon rice powder. Fry in $1\frac{1}{2}$ tablespoons ghee on a low fire and stir constantly. When fried well, add 1 tablespoon sugar, 1 tablespoon chopped almonds, and 2 tablespoons minced dates. Fry for 1–2 minutes after adding these ingredients. Eat 3–4 tablespoons every day, preferably with hot milk.

This preparation can be preserved for a week at room temperature. All preparations, where ghee is used, should not be consumed colder than the room temperature. Ghee solidifies at low temperatures and it is advised that you take it in melted form. If you store this preparation at a low temperature, keep the quantity you want to eat at room temperature for a while before eating.

---

[12] *Caraka Saṃhitā, Cikitsāsthānam*, II, (1), 47.

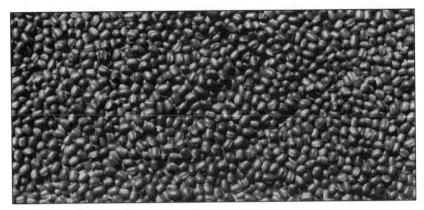

Figure 14. Urad dāl or black gram.

Another Aphrodisiac

Take ¼ cup (50 grams) each of the following: Urad dāl flour, dates, raisins, and asparagus (dried). Cook all these in about 2 quarts (2 liters) water and reduce it to one fourth. Then add 2 cups (half liter) milk and reduce the preparation to half by cooking. Add sugar according to taste. This preparation should be consumed along with boiled *śāli* rice mixed with ghee and sugar.

Yogurt Aphrodisiac

Make yogurt yourself with full cream milk as has been explained earlier. Take the upper fatty layer of this curd and add to it sugar, honey, pepper (a little), and ground cardamom. This preparation should be taken with cooked rice mixed with ghee.

Farmers' Aphrodisiac

This preparation is only possible for farmers or those who have a cow that can give milk. Nourish the cow with Urad dāl leaves or sugar cane, or leaves from the *Arjuna terminalia* tree. The cow should have a living calf. The cow should be healthy and be of a breed that gives good milk. The milk of such a cow, taken with sugar and some ghee, is an excellent aphrodisiac. If you should find such a cow, take 1½ cups of this milk and add 1 teaspoon of candy sugar (or to taste) every evening before going to bed. The same preparation is even more effective if one boils the milk for this recipe with a piece of gold or a gold ring for about 10 minutes and then takes it hot after adding some sugar and ghee. This preparation increases fertility.

Anti-Aging Aphrodisiac

Fry the fruits of long pepper *(Piper longum)* in equal quantities of ghee and sesame oil. Grind the long pepper after frying and cook it in milk-steam for half an hour. It will become like a paste. This should be taken either in small doses ($\frac{1}{2}$ teaspoon with a glass of hot milk) or with *śāli* rice cooked with milk and ghee. This preparation is particularly good for diminishing the effects of aging on sexual energy.

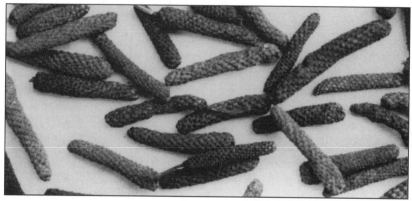

Figure 15. Long pepper.

Asparagus Aphrodisiac

Asparagus is an excellent aphrodisiac. In Āyurveda, there is a description of four kinds of asparagus. But I will not go into these details and suggest that you use the variety available in your region. If there is more than one variety available, mix them in equal quantities. Preparations of asparagus are especially good for women, and in Āyurveda, asparagus is prescribed for rejuvenating sexual energy after childbirth. Asparagus preparations are also breast promoting; they keep breasts from sagging, and are good for promoting milk. You may take either fresh or dried asparagus, but the latter should be dried in the shade and should not be more than one year old. You can make several different preparations from asparagus.

Boil the asparagus in four times their quantity of water. For example, use 2½ cups (1 kilogram) asparagus to 20 cups (4 liters) water. Cook on a low fire and reduce it to one fourth. Filter the decoction. I suggest two different preparations that can be made from this decoction.

Asparagus Ghee

Made by adding the decoction to one fourth of its quantity of ghee and then the two are cooked, uncovered, over a low fire so that all the water evaporates. In this process, the active compounds of asparagus are mixed well in the ghee. This preparation can be stored for a long time. Take ½ to 1 tablespoon daily, according to your power of digestion. Take the ghee in soup or in other hot food. For an enhanced effect, add this ghee to hot milk. You should add 1 tablespoon of ghee to 1 cup hot milk and add also 2 teaspoons sugar to it. You may add ⅛ teaspoon of either powdered black pepper or long pepper. This acts as an excellent aphrodisiac.

Asparagus Sugar Syrup

Made by adding 2 pounds (1 kilogram) sugar to 5 cups of decoction. After cooking it for about half an hour, add 1 ounce (30 grams) finely ground cardamom. Cook a little more and let cool. This syrup can be preserved for a long time. If you are in a humid place, it may get some fungus. To preserve it, cook it longer and store in a refrigerator. This syrup can be taken like a cold drink in water. Add 3 teaspoons in cold water once daily.

Increase Desire

This is a very simple preparation and its ingredients should be easy to get anywhere in the world. You need powdered licorice, ghee, honey, and milk. For one dose, mix 1 tablespoon each: powdered licorice, honey, and ghee. Whip well. You should obtain a kind of paste which should be eaten with some hot milk. It is excellent to increase the sexual urge.

To Make a Woman Happy

Fry 5 cups (1 kilogram) whole wheat flour in 1 cup (200 grams) ghee while constantly stirring. Separately, add 5 cups (1 kilogram) of candy sugar to 1¼ cups (250 ml) water and 1¼ cup ghee. Cook these until all the water is evaporated. Add this to the wheat preparation and mix them well on a low fire. It will become like a puree. When cold, add ½ pound (200 grams) honey. This preparation can be preserved for some time in cold conditions. Take 3 tablespoons or more, according to your digestive power, as a daily dose. It is said that by using this preparation, a man satisfies a woman like an elephant.

ATMOSPHERE AND RITUALS

I have talked about different forms of aphrodisiacs and other factors which promote sexual potency, vigor, etc. There are two additional factors which play an important role for enhancing sexual expression. These are the atmosphere and decor of the sleeping chamber and the importance of rituals. For sexual sharing, an appropriate atmosphere which pleases the senses and excites them (the outer atmosphere) is essential. Similarly, inner preparation or mental attitude is highly important. Following are some suggestions to that effect.

The bedroom should be airy and pleasant. It should not be overheated in winter or over-cooled in summer. It is better to cover oneself with plenty of blankets than heat the room. Over-cooled rooms are not good, as one fears exposure. Besides, the sexual act is *vāta*-promoting and so is cold.

The bedroom should be noise free as much as possible. It should smell good, but not of strong perfume. The sweet smell of jasmine, lavender, or a light incense is good. You may want to burn some aromatic herbs once a day, for this is recommended in Āyurvedic literature. The incense perfumes the room in addition to getting rid of insects and purifying the air in the room.

The bedroom should not be cluttered with too many things. It should be well-painted, clean, and orderly. The colors used in the room should be in harmony and should not be too bright and varied.

The bed should be straight, and should not sag in the middle. It should be neither too soft nor too hard. Bed sheets should not be made of synthetic material; they should be cotton or linen. Decorate the room with objects pleasing to the senses. Use some good paintings, wall hangings, or carpets with romantic scenes on them.

The room should be private. It should have doors that close and the windows should have curtains. There should be no disturbing element in the bedroom: no telephones, or any machines which make noise.

You should completely relax in this room, and not drag the day's activities to it. It is important to get rid of the hectic activity of the mind which is a usual phenomenon in our times, and slide slowly into the calmness and tranquility of the night. Many people have televisions in their bedrooms, and during a quiz show or a football game they suddenly want to "enjoy" sexual togetherness. Then they complain: "It does not work," and there are many divorces!

It is advised that prior to going to the sleeping chamber, the couple should go out for a walk, observe flowers and trees, a water source like a river or lake, or watch the moon on the moonlit nights. They should have pleasing and sweet conversation and should not get into disputes or discuss unpleasant subjects prior to retiring to their chamber. This latter can be achieved by having patience and indulgence with each other. One should make an effort to build an appropriate desire-inducing inner and outer atmosphere. It is suggested to do some breathing exercises *(prāṇāyāma)* and *śavāṣana* together (see page 121) to bring stability to the mind.

The essence of building an "inner atmosphere" for a complete and intense flow of sexual energy lies in your fundamental attitude toward sexuality. You should not think that the other person (your partner) is someone who gives you pleasure. He or she is not an object of pleasure for you, like a good meal or your possessions. Even if you are thinking of sexual pleasure, it is you, yourself, who create that pleasure for yourself. Sexuality is much more than driving pleasure. It is sharing and merging two complementary energies into each other, and it is blissful. During sexual union, you should try to distance yourself from the material world. In addition, for a blissful sexual experience, you should have respect for each other. It is not only the respect for someone's ideas or body or any other feature, but a profound respect for the other person's whole being. Try to see in each other not only the flesh and blood and other external and personality features, but the deeper and more profound part. This latter is not the material substance of a person.

Visualize a flame symbolic of energy in the other person. Visualize the same flame within yourself. Then "see" the two flames come closer and closer and merge into each other. Their merging will give rise to a very strong light. In this big envelope of light is all the phenomenal world—children, parents, trains, cars, flowers, trees, birds, lakes, all that exists. This merging signifies cosmic creation. The sexual union is symbolic of the union of *Puruṣa* (the Universal Soul) with the *Prakṛti* (the Cosmic Substance). It is this union which is the cause of this phenomenal world and our being on this Earth. Thus, through a sexual union, you are symbolizing the cosmic creation.[13] It is sacred; it is holy. For arriving at this realization, you have to slowly transcend the physical to cause the merging of the two inner energies. To transcend the physical, you have to live intensely, and that is done by enhancing your sensuality. We have already discussed this subject.

It is also important to learn that you can slowly, with small rituals, go through this intense realization of the physical. For example, this may be done by anointing each other's body with sandalwood paste. You should look at the details of the body while doing this ceremony, and enjoy the beauty, complexity, and vastness of the human form. The same can be done by many other methods, like touching each and every part of the body with a sweet smelling flower, with light massage, or just intense visualization. For this latter, you may do *śavāsana* (see page 121) together and after visualizing and concentrating on your own body, do the same for that of your partner. You should also include in this visualization the details of each other's sex organs in addition to what has been already described for this āsana. This, however, does not mean that you should over-imagine and lose your direction. In this ceremony, you are only concentrating on the parts to enjoy their beauty and not for "sexual pleasure." For some of you, doing this successfully may need considerable mental effort.

I will not go into the details of the various ceremonies and rituals as readers have their own rituals and traditions. In India, we believe that these things one knows without even learning them

---

[13] For details of the concept of *Puruṣa* and *Prakṛti*, see my book, *Patañjali's Yoga Sūtras: A Scientific Exposition* (New Delhi: Clarion Books, 1993).

from parents or other people, as they are passed from generation to generation with a subtle energy (which is beyond the scope of modern research in genetics).[14] Sometimes grandparents observing their 2-year old grandchild remark: "Oh, he is doing exactly what his father did when he was 2 years old." You see that babies do many things their parents did without being taught to do so. This is what I mean by the subtle energy being passed on from generation to generation. It also brings us our heritage in the field of sexuality. However, with unnatural ways of living and losing track of the cosmic rhythm, we also lose our cultural heritage. The above descriptions will initiate you in this direction, and by concentrating the mind, you will also invent your own ways and ceremonies. I have described the fundamentals, and the most essential is to learn to achieve stillness of mind and concentrate your mental energy to evoke sexual energy from every pore in your body.

SOME COMMONLY OCCURRING SEXUAL PROBLEMS

This is a very extensive theme and is dealt with in my specific books on women and men.[15] However, I will discuss very briefly some common problems and their possible treatment.

Impotence

Impotence may have multiple causes in different age groups. In some young men, inhibition and the fear of facing a woman may cause it. An encounter with a tough and challenging woman who lacks the qualities of motherhood[16] for a first sexual interaction may

---

[14] For modern concepts in this field, see Rupert Sheldrake's book, *The Rebirth of Nature* (London: Century, 1990).

[15] *Kamasūtra for Women* was published in German, and will be published in English by Kodansha. I am also in the process of writing a book on Āyurvedic wisdom for men.

[16] See my book *Kamasūtra for Women* for a detailed description of the concept of motherhood.

give rise to the problem of temporary impotence. Appropriate and timely help, in the form of consultations, and an encounter and relationship with an experienced, older, tender-hearted woman may easily cure this problem. Knowing the problem, the woman should lead the man step by step, with words of consolation and reassurance, thus restoring his lost confidence. As a woman, you should not be impatient or give up on these men, as once they are cured of their initial inhibition, they may turn out to be very virile and talented in this dimension of their being.

Impotency due to aging can be easily cured by taking the appropriate aphrodisiacs (see Anti-Aging Aphrodisiac, page 89). Impotency may also be caused because of general weakness or fatigue conditions. When *ojas* (vitality and immunity) is low, like other vital functions of the body, sexuality is also affected. Rejuvenating products, a balanced and unctuous diet, and some aphrodisiacs will cure this problem. However, before these treatments, it is essential to create an equilibrium in the body's humors. Inner cleaning practices *(panchakarma)* should be done, and bodily fire (digestion) should be in order. Otherwise, the intake of rejuvenating products and aphrodisiacs will be wasted, as they are not well assimilated in the body.

Impotence is a *vāta* disorder. This imbalance may be caused by various factors, such as fear, nervousness, the lack of sleep or appropriate rest, nutrition imbalance, constipation, etc., and these should be immediately attended to.

Lastly, you should be aware that impotence may also be caused due to the side-effects of some chemical drugs. Without going into the details of such drugs, I would advise that if you are taking any drug regularly and simultaneously notice any change in your sexuality, do try to find out the details of the side-effects of that drug.

Premature Ejaculation

For the complete fulfillment of both partners, it is essential that the sexual duration of both partners is in accord. Some men have a problem with premature ejaculation. Since women require a relatively longer time to reach the peak of their sexual expression, this becomes a serious sexual problem for men. Again, this is a *vāta* ailment and you should emphasize balancing this humor.[17] Try to attain a peaceful mental state through yoga and concentration practices, and also make sure that you get peaceful and tranquil sleep. Follow some of the instructions given in Part III to this effect. *Panchakarma* practices (five practices for inner cleaning) are highly recommended to purify the body. Then try some rejuvenating and aphrodisiac products. A few recipes to enhance the power of retention follow.

Retention Power Number 1

Put a pinch of camphor in $\frac{1}{8}$ cup (25 ml) rose essence and mix well. Apply this on the penis in a very small quantity by putting 2–3 drops of it on your fingers and then smearing it on penis about an hour before intercourse.

Retention Power Number 2

Powdered root of *Basilicum sanctum* can be made into a fine paste. Grind in a mortar and add water. This can be applied to the penis about an hour before intercourse to enhance retention and vigor.

Retention Power Number 3

Take 1 ounce (25 grams) each of cinnamon, pepper, cardamom, nutmeg, mace (aril of nutmeg seeds called *Javitri* in Hindi), pine nuts, dried ginger, cloves, and dried coconut. Grind all of these into a fine powder. Add to this $\frac{1}{2}$ ounce (12 grams) powdered saffron, and mix well. Mix all this gradually with honey, just enough to make a thick paste so that you are able to make pills from it. Make chickpea-sized pills. Take 3 to 4 of these pills (or $\frac{1}{4}$ teaspoon if you did not make pills) daily with hot milk or tea. Take this treatment for 20 to 40 days. This enhances sexual vigor and retention, and also cures impotence in some cases.

Lack of Vaginal Secretions

If a woman does not have sexual secretions (or *kamajal* as it is called in Sanskrit) with sexual activity, either she is suffering from *vāta* or she has a mental block or is inhibited. Sexual expression is a natural urge, like the other urges of hunger, thirst, urine,

---

[17] For details see *Ayurveda: A Way of Life,* also published by Samuel Weiser.

stool, etc. It is generally observed that women who have this problem are also suffering from allied problems, like constipation, irregular menstruation, or other inhibitions in expressing themselves. To cure this problem, in addition to doing some physical treatments, a woman should undergo a holistic check up. Sexual secretions are also blocked when a woman is with a man whom she does not trust, or does not really love, or she is thinking of another man, or having feelings of guilt. This problem also occurs when she finds her partner not tender and indulgent enough. Thus, it is very important to find the root cause of the problem.

It is recommended to do the breathing exercises and to purify the energy channels, as the site of the *kamajala* is the moon channel (see Part III).

Some women have difficulty reaching the peak of their sexual expression, commonly termed orgasm. In some cases it happens simply because they need more time and the partner has a shorter retention period. In this case, two measures can be taken. First, the man can follow the above-described recipes to enhance his retention period, and second, the woman can take measures to shorten the time she needs. As has been described previously, she should develop her sensuous capacities and enhance the power of her concentration. During the sexual act, she should devote her mental and physical power completely to evoking her dormant sexual energy (for details refer to *Kamasūtra for Women*).

Taking aphrodisiacs, or adding them to your food, enhances sexual energy and facilitates achieving sexual fulfillment. You may regularly use ginger, garlic, pepper, long pepper, and nutmeg in your cooking. Eating unctuous food and avoiding *vāta*-enhancing products is also recommended.

In the folk tradition of some parts of India, women smear their vagina to enhance the rapidity of orgasm. The products used are a pinch of boric acid, or camphor, mixed with honey; or tamarind fruit pulp mixed with honey and a pinch of pepper.[18]

---

[18] Readers should note that I do not recommend that you try these folk remedies, as you may have allergies that you have not checked out. Pure blood and good health are important to attain first. If you try any of these methods, you do so of your own volition.

OTHER ASPECTS OF SEXUALITY

Sexual Desire

The reader must be clear on the term "sexual desire," which I use during the course of this book. Sexual desire is different from the desire for sex. Sexual desire is not something which is in your imagination. It is not like having a desire for worldly things. It should be differentiated from worldly desires. In this latter context, it will be the "desire for sex." For example, someone may fantasize about his "sexual desires." One may desire to have someone special as sex partner; or may desire a particular sexual relationship in special circumstances, etc. When I talk about sexual desire, it is a complex psycho-physical response of our being which gives rise to a compelling force within us. This compelling force is the cause of the continuity of the phenomenal world.

It is important to differentiate between desire for sex and "sexual desire" as many people waste sexual energy because of an excessive desire for sex. They think too much about this part of life, and when there is time for the "sexual desire," they lack physiological and mental expression. It is essential to have self-control regarding one's desires for sex in order to enhance sexual energy.

The world is full of temptations. One must learn to have limitations not only in practice, but also in one's imagination. There are always more beautiful men or women than your partner. Appreciate what you have.

Body, Mind and Sexuality

Āyurvedic sages were well aware that the seat of sexual behavior and energy is both mind and body.

> Potency is based upon sexual exhilaration, which again depends upon the strength of body and mind.[19]

Strength of both body and mind is very important for complete sexual exhilaration and expression. For developing strength of

---

[19] *Caraka Saṃhitā, Cikitsāsthānam*, II, (4), 43–45.

mind, we need to begin with the body, to get to know its activities, and to be aware of changes due to environment, time, weather, social change, etc. The next step is to learn about our cosmic link through *prāṇāyāma*, the yogic practices for breathing. Finally, we must try to learn concentration practices (popularly, but incorrectly, called meditation).[20] Besides these practices, strength of mind lies in assimilating good qualities, such as kindness, humility, patience, being contented with our circumstances, detachment, and the lack of greed or anger. These qualities provide us with strength of mind and character, and give us an attractive and radiant look. These features are essential for looking sexually attractive and desirable. In yogic literature, it is said that a yogi acquires a radiant and sexually attractive look when he has assimilated good qualities, such as friendship, non-violence, etc.[21] However, worldly people (who are not ascetics and who live normal family lives) cannot be compared to yogis and ascetics. This example only demonstrates that, with strength of mind and character, we can look attractive because of our inner state.

No two human beings look alike. Even identical twins can be differentiated by their mother. Just as human beings vary in their outward appearance, similarly, they differ in their personalities and sexual behavior. For an unrestricted flow of sexual energy, one should be indulgent, understanding, patient, and selfless with one's partner. One should not think of proving one's great potency and vigor without paying attention to the reactions of the partner.

Patience and tolerance are important qualities for enhancing sexual vigor and energy. These qualities are important, not only in relation to one's partner, but as a general social attitude. It is observed that many people blame others for their problems. They use all their energy in grumbling. For example, they blame their sexual problems on their childhood, parents, or other circumstances in their lives.[22] It is useless to blame others for things

---

[20] For a clarification on the subject of meditation, the reader may refer to my book, *Patañjali's Yoga Sūtras*.

[21] See *Patañjali's Yoga Sūtras*.

[22] Modern psychology and social sciences have done tremendous harm in this direction. It is observed that young people all over the world tend to acquire an attitude of blaming others for their problems. The special victims in this direction are the parents. It is always very convenient and comfortable to shed off your responsibility and find a "rationale" for it.

which have been already done, as it is impossible to go back to those events in the same circumstances. Instead of blaming and grumbling, one should put the energy into improving upon the situation. Forget, forgive, and be constructive.

You should learn from the past, but not live in the past. You should think of ways to improve your present difficulties and problems. Improve upon what you are, what your parents were, and what you inherited from them. Past *karma* is already done. Present *karma* is the most important for improving upon the past and for building a better future. If you have problems related to sexuality, take them as a challenge and be determined to get rid of them. You should put your will and energy into that. You may trace the origin of your problems, in order to get rid of them, but not for blaming others. For example, if you know that you have a certain problematic behavior because of some incident in your childhood, you should tell yourself: "Well, it is good that I know where my problem originates, but now I must concentrate on getting rid of it. The shadow of the past should not accompany me. I am determined to get rid of the effect of past troubles, and I will use my will and might for it."

This constructive attitude will open way for the present and future sexual bliss. Live in the present moment and rebuild it, even if you have "ruins" from the past.

Sexual energy is intensified with companionship and sharing joys and sorrows of life. What gives strength to a relationship is sharing the pains and perils. Some people look at sexuality and companionship in a fragmented way. Sexuality is associated with joy. At difficult and painful moments, they prefer to be alone. They do not like to share their grief with their partner, and somehow wish to escape showing the other a grief-stricken, non-energetic, and dull aspect of their existence. This is particularly true in Western culture. A relationship never becomes profound with this attitude. Sharing life events only partially gives rise to a restricted flow of sexual energy between the two individuals. I do not deny that the sensuous pleasure is there, but what I mean to convey is that without complete sharing, one can not achieve an experience of bliss which is at a much more elevated level than the physical. I have also described a method of using this intense sexual energy for healing in the next section.

In the beginning of this book, I talked about both the reductionist and the holistic approach to medicine. In the present context of sexuality, unlike the modern medicine, Āyurveda does not believe that sexual excretions are limited to their physiological sites. It is said that they are diffused "all over the sentient body, as juice in sugar cane, *ghee* in curd,[23] and oil in sesame seeds. The sexual secretions discharged in man and woman during sexual activity flow like water from a wet cloth because of pressure, action, and determination. Exhilaration, sexual desire, movement, sliminess, pressure, subtlety, and the impulse of *vāta* are factors leading to the discharge of sexual excretions from the body, which are known as the material substratum of the moving and omnipresent soul."[24]

Āyurveda lays great emphasis on the relationship of body, mind, and soul, and the relationship of soul with cosmic energy. I want to discuss this concept in the context of sexual energy. Let us begin with the material substratum of the soul—the body—the seat of sensuous pleasure. You must keep in mind that the sex organs and other sensitive areas of concentrated sexual energy are not the only areas that provide exhilaration. Each and every part of the body has an intense store of sexual energy that remains dormant because of our social or cultural conditioning. Sensuality is evoked with practice and experience. This subject has been already partially discussed in the section on enhancing sensuous power. Furthermore, all parts of the body should be included in sexual sharing for both exhilaration and fulfillment. The soles of the feet, the spaces between the fingers, the sides of the hands and feet, the sides of the waist—all should be involved to get the most tactile sensation. Simultaneous use of the other senses should also not be ignored. Hearing gentle words of appreciation in an appropriate atmosphere is highly desire provoking. To enhance, as well as prolong, sexual exhilaration, it is essential to be completely involved in your actions. You should make every effort to concentrate; to be there with body, mind, and soul. This means that you get totally involved with your activities, forgetting about the external world, problems, fears, anxieties, and the unknown future. Be there in your entirety. The two persons involved in sexual sharing should express themselves unhindered in every re-

---

[23] In India, the traditional method of making butter which gives rise to *ghee* is by churning the yogurt.

[24] *Caraka Saṃhitā, Cikitsāsthānam,* II, (4), 46–49.

spect, in order to have an experience of oneness of the two energies, and the realization of the human link with the cosmos.

We humans, with our day-to-day worldly existence, are too much involved with sensory perception. Most of us feel that whatever we perceive from the senses and cognize by the mind is the only reality. We forget the power (śakti) which makes the phenomenal world possible. We are somehow conditioned to only recognize material reality. All of us experience the reality beyond sensory perception, but we ignore it, or call it a delusion, or think its a paranormal experience. Through sexuality, we have a similar experience, for we transcend our senses momentarily. Most people confuse this experience with the joy of senses. The reason for this is ignorance. The moment of stillness, the peak of sexual interaction, is very brief. Transcendence of senses, experience of immensity, and return again to the phenomenal world happens too rapidly for a complete realization of that experience. Our purpose in the present context is to learn to prolong the moment of stillness, and to enjoy that bliss which is beyond any worldly bliss we have known. This intense energy can also be channeled for several other useful purposes, like healing, making predictions, and enhancing intuitive knowledge. In other words, with this intense sexual energy, we can develop extrasensory perception.

The paranormal ability, psychic phenomena, and the attainment of other extraordinary powers have the same fundamental basis as described above. They are also attained by transcending phenomenal reality and entering into a larger cosmic reality. The methods used for this purpose are diverse. One may use yogic ways, sexuality, or other techniques, but the fundamental basis is to transcend the senses and reach cosmic immensity. For transcending the senses, we need to learn to control the mind. The mind is controlled by the mind, itself. Through breathing and concentration practices, the stillness of the mind is achieved. When the mind gets free from a constant chain of thoughts, it becomes a part of the soul, which, in turn, is part of cosmic energy and is not involved with the phenomenal world.

I have described many preparatory methods for attaining a blissful sexual experience. I do not want to go into too many details for two reasons. First, there is no prescribed formula, as people are so varied and creative. Techniques are developed there and then, spontaneously according to time, need, and compatibility. I have described certain fundamentals which will make a solid foundation. You can construct and create in your own way and style. Second, if I describe too many techniques telling you how to prolong the moment of sexual bliss and immensity, you may get lost in the techniques themselves and never reach the destination.

In essence, you must know that the Āyurvedic way of life is a prerequisite for reaching your destination. You need a healthy body and mind. Then you need to learn to control your mind, acquire good character, and use breathing techniques. Breathing is absolutely essential, as it helps control the mind and is important for increasing sexual vigor. Besides, for prolonging the bliss of sexual experience, one needs to practice breath control. During the sexual act, one goes through various phases—activity, extreme activity, stillness, and listlessness. They are all well marked by diverse breathing. *Prāṇāyāma* practices help develop control over all these steps. At the peak of sexual experience, when one transcends the sensuous, one should prolong this blissful moment by controlling the breath. This, however, can only be achieved when you have attained a long time experience in prolonging the moment of holding the vital air inside you, and holding the lungs without air.

During the prolonged experience of sexual bliss, time acquires another dimension. Time in Āyurveda, and also in the yogic tradition, is defined as the change from one moment to another. "Moment" here signifies something like a millisecond. This quality of change belongs to matter only. So, time has significance only in phenomenal reality. When we transcend the phenomenal world, which we perceive through the senses and mind, and become one with cosmic energy, there is no change and no time. There is only stillness and bliss which is beyond description.

Before closing this section, I wish to add a few words for my readers in the West. Western minds are accustomed to categorize and compartmentalize. Materialism, sensuality, sexuality, spirituality—all these are classified and categorized. In Indian thinking, whether it is medicine, speculation about reality (like yoga, *Sāṃkhya, Vedānta*, etc.) or sexuality (see the *Kāmasūtra* and other Indian literature on this subject), they are all blended together, and represent cosmic reality at different levels. Many Western historians, when talking about India, make the mistake of compartmentalizing Indian tradition into various phases of materialism, spirituality, asceticism, etc. They all existed simultaneously, and one does not deny the other; they are all shades of reality. However, the Hindu tradition maintains that sensory reality is only a tiny part of the gross cosmic reality. There are layers and layers of reality that submerge into each other, like a spiral.

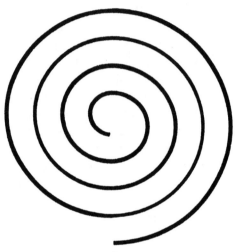

Figure 16. The spiral.

PART III

ĀYURVEDIC HEALING METHODS

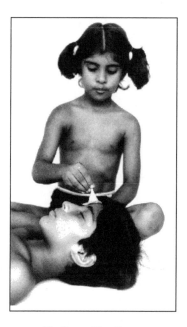

Healing with a flower.

Oh pain-giving fever, you are born out of that fire in which the wise and the righteous make offerings. You are rendering life difficult. Upon sprinkling hot water, you leave all parts of the body and go away to be dissolved in your originator, which is fire.

Athārva Veda, I, 25, 1.
1500 B.C.

5

FUNDAMENTALS
OF HEALING

L ET ME BEGIN BY EXPLAINING what is meant by "healing" in the present context, as it can be quite easily misunderstood. The word "healer" (one who has capacity to heal) has many different usages. A healer may be one who puts his hand on an ailing person and the person is cured. A healer may also be one who helps in the process of healing by doing a light massage, or using some other method of working with the body and mind. Similarly, certain places of worship, some water sources associated with these places, certain special holy trees, mountains, etc., are known to have healing energy.

First of all, you must know that it is the body which has an inbuilt capacity to heal itself. When we speak of the body in Āyurveda, it always includes mind. The total human form is taken into consideration. For example, when you get a little cut on your finger, it gets healed in the course of time. It happens by the process of regeneration of the cells. The wounded cells are replaced by new cells. The damaged cells die, and are thrown out in the form of pus. When the wound is slightly bigger, it needs to be cured with some ointment. The function of the ointment is to save the wound from infection, and to create a congenial atmosphere for the regenerating cells. It is not the ointment which does the actual healing. The new cells have to be formed to replace the old damaged ones, and the old cells have to be thrown out as debris. The purpose of medication, physicians, healing methods, and other medical aids is to help enhance the body's process of healing, and to lessen the suffering. Therefore, "healing" in the present context refers to the effort to quicken the process of cure, to use the capacity of the mind and the inner energy (soul) to be with the ailing part and strengthen it. When you are able to concentrate your mind, regulate the process of breathing, and establish a connection with the inner immense energy, you are able to heal yourself and others.

Healing reestablishes the body's energy with the cosmic rhythm in order to enhance the body's regenerating capacity, and to attain humoral harmony (the equilibrium of *vāta*, *pitta*, and *kapha*). The methods of healing discussed are not exclusive of appropriate nutrition, timely and correct medical assistance, or other means of cure. They are in addition to all the Āyurvedic health care practices described earlier.[1, 2] If you are using only healing methods, and otherwise leading an anti-health life by eating poorly, not sleeping enough, leading a sedentary life, having an excessively hectic routine, you will not be very successful with the healing methods. What I want to convey is that the Āyurvedic way of life includes healing methods meant to aid recovery, to minimize suffering, and to maintain health or prevent ailments. They are principally based upon developing consciousness of the energy that is the cause of being (Universal Energy)[3] and to radiate that inner energy in each part of the body.

Energy is invisible; it is without substance. Cosmic Substance is pervaded by the Cosmic Energy or the Universal Soul. The combination of substance and energy makes the phenomenal world. This invisible energy is everywhere and is in everything. It is this energy that is responsible for the movements of an atom to Earth rotation. It pervades plants, animals, stones, rivers, earth, wind, and all that is. Healing goes beyond substance, and establishes a connection with Cosmic Energy. It reestablishes disturbed, obstructed, or lost harmony. The disharmony could be in our

---

[1] V. Verma, 1991, *Yoga for Integral Health* (New Delhi: Hind Pocket Books, 1991).

[2] V. Verma *Ayurveda: A Way of Life* (York Beach, ME: Samuel Weiser, 1995).

[3] Universal Energy or Cosmic Energy is that energy which puts life into the Cosmic Substance. It is the combination of these two which makes the phenomenal world. Cosmic Substance is lifeless and inert and cannot act. Cosmic Energy has no substance and it cannot act. When these two combine, life and action begin. In our being, soul is the part of the Cosmic Energy, whereas our body belongs to the Cosmic Substance. This theory is from the *Sāṃkhya darśana*, one of the six schools of speculative thought in the Hindu tradition. The *Sāṃkhya darśana* forms the philosophical basis of both Yoga and Āyurveda. For details, see my book, *The Yoga Sūtras of Patañjali: A Scientific Exposition* (New Delhi: Clarion Books, 1993), or consult the original *Saṃkhya* literature.

inner and outer environment; the inner environment consists of the body, mind, and the relationship between the two. The outer environment is the social, climatic, geographical, cosmic environment. Attaining consciousness of the inner and outer environments is the first step in healing. The second step is to develop the power of the mind to realize the power of the self *(ātmaśakti)* and to use it for balancing deranged harmony.

GENERAL INSTRUCTIONS FOR HEALING

If you want to learn to heal, whether yourself or others, you must begin by working on yourself. Use the following basic concepts and assumptions.

1. The human body is not a machine. I have already discussed this topic in the introduction. Modern people think that the body functions like a machine because of the influence of contemporary medicine, and because technologically advanced societies work like mechanical systems. We cannot learn healing methods if we remain in the narrow framework of these mechanistic views. The holistic view of life is contrary to the mechanistic view. It considers cosmos a constantly changing dynamic whole, where everything is interlinked and interdependent. It is the interlink and the interdependence between the fundamental cosmic energies which is the basis of healing. In the mechanistic view, on the other hand, the universe works like a machine and so do our bodies.

Modern medicine is based upon a mechanistic view; the various mechanisms of the body are understood at biological and molecular levels, and an illness is viewed as a malfunctioning of the parts of the body-machine. An illness is treated by physical and/or chemical intervention. Therefore, the talk of inner power, Cosmic Energy, and using all this to enhance the process of healing and recovery is ridiculous from the point of view of modern medicine. In order to illustrate what I mean in reference to healing, the following example demonstrates how the holistic approach of Āyurveda is different from the mechanistic and reductionist approach.

Imagine someone who has frequent headaches, who goes to a physician known to practice modern medicine. This person is given painkillers to handle the pain. Perhaps the eyes are tested to make sure the pain does not originate there. If there is also a complaint of disturbed sleep, some sedatives may also be given. Usually, nutrition, the person's social and spiritual aspects, and other environmental factors are not taken into consideration. If this person does not get cured with the given treatment, he or she is referred to a neurologist, where further tests, like computer tomography, blood tests for any possible virus, or other parasites, in his or her brain are made. If no cause for the headache is found, this person is referred to psychiatry. There, for the first time, this person's illness is viewed in its mental and social context. The allopathic doctors may even infer that the illness is psychosomatic.

In Āyurveda, a person is not treated in fragments as in the above description. In holistic medicine, a person cannot be reduced to parts. When this same person with a headache goes to see an Āyurvedic physician, the following data are requested: details of evacuation, digestion, constipation, nutrition, the familial situation, and social circumstances. The cause of the headache is not considered to be localized only in the head. The frequent headaches may occur due to constipation, stomach acidity, some posture defects of the neck, a blocked nose, or other allied breathing problems. They could also be due to a nutritional imbalance ultimately related to stomach problems. They could also be caused by fear and tension that affects the breathing process and increases *vāta* in the body. The excessive *vāta* may also give rise to disturbed sleep or insomnia. In Āyurveda, the job of the physician is to find the fundamental causes of the ailments and eradicate them with various therapeutical measures.

There are three types of therapies in Āyurveda: rational, psychological, and spiritual. Healing, the method we are presently concerned with, comes in the third category. Spiritual, in the present context, refers to the inner energy, or *ātmaśakti* (let us call it spiritual energy). Our spiritual energy is pure and immortal, and is a part of the immense Cosmic Energy. By evoking this energy through concentration (or meditation) practices, we establish our link to the immense Universal Energy which can be used for healing.

    2. We humans are capable of enhancing our sensuality with Āyurveda. We can enhance the use of our senses with conscious effort. This does not mean that we learn only to enjoy more with our senses; it means that we widen the experience of our senses to develop an extraordinary sensibility (see also Part II). It also includes something new, something which we may dislike and reject with fear. For example, when something is bitter to taste, people find it awful. Their minds work with some established notion of sweet and salty being good, and bitter being bad. To enhance sensuality, we must savor *all* in life. I do not mean merely different *rasas*,[4] but life in all its dimensions. This widens our mental capabilities through experience and gives us a keen sense of observation in relation to the body. An enhanced sensibility is very helpful for detecting ailments from their rudimentary and subjective symptoms, so we can provide timely help. We can also use various healing methods to avoid the sickness "not yet come." This is an old concept in Āyurveda; today it is beginning to be considered in the West: it is called preventive medicine. But with all the preventive techniques, few Westerners use the techniques I present here.

    3. Each part of the human body is equally important. All parts of the body are holy and sacred, and hence worthy of respect. You must make sure that each part of your body is well-nourished. Your duty is not only to appease the fire of your stomach and to satisfy the urges; it is important to nourish every part of your body with energy. For that, you should make sure that all the energy channels are open. According to Āyurveda, when *kapha* accumulates in certain parts of the body, the channels are closed and that part of the body is not well-nourished. When this state is maintained over a long period of time, a disease develops. With the enhanced sensitivity, and with the help of some yogic practices, one

---

[4] It is not possible to translate the word *rasa*. In Āyurvedic language, the classification of drugs is based upon their *rasas*. The literal meaning of the word *rasa* is "juice," or "taste," or "essence." Although drugs are classified as bitter, sweet, astringent, etc., *rasa* signifies much more than taste. It signifies the complete sensual experience and the total effect of that substance with that particular taste. Our tongue qualifies the taste, but when the substance enters into our body, it has multiple effects on us. The basis of this classification is that tastes, and their effects on us, are related. *Rasas* are further related to the humors. For details, see my book *Ayurveda: A Way of Life.*

is able to detect imbalances and can take steps to reestablish the lost harmony.

4. *The inner energy and the power we have talked about is not only to be used to heal the ailing parts, but we also must learn to use this energy to maintain a state of health.* We have to learn to make an armor *(kavacha)* of this energy around ourselves to protect ourselves from external attacks of any kind. In Āyurveda, we do not consider that a disease is only limited to the physical ailments of the body. If we are afraid of a situation or a person, if we feel discouraged, or are greedy, jealous, or have any other mind disturbing attribute, it shows an unhealthy state. We also must learn to protect ourselves from these qualities of mind, as they are the cause of many serious diseases. To cure a negative mental attitude through healing ceremonies is a very ancient Āyurvedic practice, and we will come to this subject in detail a little later.

All this may sound very complicated and difficult at this stage. Indeed, to evoke your inner power, you need to make tremendous effort in the beginning. The time and effort required to achieve this goal will also vary from person to person. Relatively quiet people, who are not restless and are able to concentrate easily, will need less time than those who are agile, talkative, and nervous.

To put this in simple words, if you want to learn how to heal, first you have to develop your intuitive capacity. Guided by this intuitive capacity, you will have to diagnose the root cause of your ailment and then enhance the process of healing by consolation, encouragement, and by providing extra energy to the ailing part. Actually, all living beings have a natural gift of finding their troubles and acting accordingly, so that they are rapidly healed and do not suffer. This gift springs out of the innate desire of all living beings to remain alive and to save themselves from death and suffering. However, in humans, the capacity to establish harmony within ourselves (and with nature) has been lost, due to our conditioning and life circumstances. Animals are healthier than we are; they cure themselves without doctors and hospitals; their apothecary is Mother Nature, herself. When we carefully watch animals in nature (not domestic animals), we find no obese frogs, birds, or rabbits. They know how to keep an equilibrium between food and activities. Similarly, they have an intuitive power to be selective in their nutrition for curing themselves. They have no social security or health insurance, or other means to depend upon for keeping good health. Therefore, their strength lies within themselves. They use their inner energy to heal themselves. Of course there are several diseases animals suffer from. It is observed that human beings are largely responsible for the big troubles animals have. Human beings disturb the ecological balance, which hinders the harmony between animals and nature, and this becomes a cause of illness, and even extinction.

People who have healing capacities to use for themselves, or for healing others, are like any one of you. Basically you have the same capability, but this energy lies dormant in you. Awakening this energy is possible; it needs a strong sense of goal, perseverance, and discipline.

PRACTICAL ASPECTS OF HEALING

I will explain the healing methods in very simple steps so that you find it easy to achieve your goal.

Developing an "I" and "You" Relationship with the Body

In an orchestra, the role of the conductor is very important. It is a role that coordinates people so they can play harmoniously. A good conductor knows his team, their talents, and is sensitive to all the sounds of the different instruments. It is this sensitivity which qualifies a conductor. In the context of healing, you are the orchestra conductor, and you have to develop an awareness and sensitivity about each and every part of your body. Each part of your body has an individual identity and function, and at the same time, all these parts form an integral part of the whole. The coordination of the functions of various parts with each other is absolutely essential for maintaining a harmony with the whole. You must learn to treat each part of your body as if it has an individual identity. Remember always that different parts of your body are dynamic organisms which have a capacity to regenerate. They are not the parts of a non-living machine that can be replaced when they break. You must learn to recognize their identity and develop a relationship with each one.

When a child gets hurt, the spontaneous reaction of the mother is to be protective and consoling; healing the child with love is as necessary as first aid. You have to develop the same attitude of love, protection, and care toward the individual parts of your body. This love should not be in the form of self-indulgence, but a genuine feeling from the depth of your heart. Love, consideration, and care are primary qualities you need for learning to heal. For attaining these qualities, you have to get rid of the negative qualities, such as jealousy, selfishness, competition, and anger. We all have immense love within us, which is covered with the dust of our negative attributes. Methods to get rid of these negative qualities are discussed later.

Let us do a practical exercise so that these ideas become clear.

Situation: A persisting pain in the right ankle. No apparent cause is known to you. Normally, in such a situation, you will treat the ailing part with warm therapy, pain-relieving oil or ointment, and other measures in this direction. All these are a part of rational therapy. The first part of healing is that the physical handling and treatment should be done as if your ankle, your foot, and that whole ailing area is like a small helpless baby who needs your help. You should give this area a light healing massage and keep it covered to save it from exposure. With love and care, you need to develop a relationship with this part of your body and should be able to talk to it. You should tell this part its vital importance for you. You should ask your foot something like this: "Tell me, what is wrong with you? Tell me the cause of your trouble? Please do not stay sick too long. You see, you form the base for the rest of me. I cannot walk without your cooperation. Are you angry with me because I misused you? Did I not take enough care of you? Was I standing too long without balancing the weight on two of you? Was I making a tense posture with you?" etc.

While talking like this to a part of your body, you will slowly learn to bring to the surface all the possible problems which may have caused the ailment or disorder. You will also attain consciousness about the ailing part, and you will start to pay special attention to it all the time. You will discover the cause of your problem. You will see that slowly, that particular part of your body will also begin to talk to you. You will feel that you have rediscovered yourself. Obviously, the "talking" will be an intuitive communication. You will be becoming sensual—and aware.

Let me tell you of my own experience to illustrate my statement. Several years ago, I started to have pain in my right shoulder. Since it was winter, I thought that the pain was due to an exposure to cold. I took all precautions and regularly put pain-relieving oil on my shoulder. The pain was under control, but it was recurring. This persisting pain was slowly spreading to my neck and arm. I felt that gradually it was becoming chronic. I believe that nothing exists without a cause, and when a pain persists, its causes should be thoroughly investigated and removed before it is too late. I seriously started to investigate the causes of this pain with the above-described methods. I used to work long hours; I was writing a lot at this time. My various conversations with the ailing part revealed the cause of this pain. The story was the following: in the process of writing, I was obviously using the muscles of the right hand, arm, and shoulder. But what I discovered was that I was also writing when I was not writing. That means that I was keeping my fingers in a tense posture of holding a pen. In fact, this process was more stressful than the process of writing. I even discovered that my right hand was in a writing posture when I woke up from sleep. After obtaining this knowledge, it was easy to cure myself. First, I made a conscious effort to check that my fingers, hand, and arm were not tensed when I was not writing. Second, I tried to go deeper into the cause of this problem of writing when I was not writing. It was my deep-seated desire to be more productive than I was. This was perhaps the reason that I kept writing in my sleep. There was a mental state of dissatisfaction and greed that was ultimately responsible for my trouble. The lack of satisfaction gives rise to greed and the greed may be for anything.

I have told this story to demonstrate that a search within ourselves can save us from a lot of health hazards. Imagine somebody with the same problem of pain, but this person does not believe in holistic methods of cure and therefore does not take any responsibility for curing herself or himself. This person thinks that a doctor can cure this problem, and goes to an allopathic physician. The patient is given ointments, pain-relieving tablets, etc., as an immediate measure to combat pain. The ailing part will be X-rayed; the patient may also be given a blood test. When the reports show nothing about the cause of pain, the patient is advised to continue with pain-relieving tablets, ointment, physiotherapy, etc. In this process, this person may become more sick than before because of the side-effects of the pain-relieving pills. If the pain persists over a long period of time, the patient is told that the cause of the pain is perhaps in his or her mind, and is referred to psychiatry. Thus, there is a strict division between the ailments of the body and the problems of the mind. There are many people in this world who suffer from chronic pains of an unknown origin. Many of these suffering individuals are relatively young, and they have to learn to live with their pain as modern medicine does not provide an appropriate cure for such troubles. Some typical examples of pains of unknown origin are in the following regions: wrist, thumb, arm, shoulder, neck, other parts of the back, knee, ankle, or leg.

Sometimes, you may not be able to find the cause of your pain yourself, and you may need external help. You should also remember that the methods of healing described here are not exclusive of other therapeutic measures, such as the application of heat, oil, massage (rational therapy). As has been said earlier, in Āyurveda, the three types of therapies are described, the other two being psychological and spiritual. Methods described here include both psychological and spiritual therapy. It is only by a simultaneous application of these three methods that it becomes possible to cure small but nagging pains.

When you develop an "I" and "you" relationship with different parts of your body, you will see that, slowly, a beautiful communication will be there between you and them, and "you" will be no more your mind alone. This will lead you to stop exploiting your body and misusing it. You will begin to listen to its needs and complaints. For example, if you have a habit of dragging yourself for outings despite a headache or some other discomfort, you will begin to pause and think about it. You will also begin to avoid those tempting eatables which, once inside you, create upheaval. This self-aware way of being will give good results, and your minor problems will be handled by you before they become big.

No serious health problem or disease appears in a day. We make enough ground for a big ailment to be there. By healing small ailments as soon as they arise, or even before they arise, we save ourselves from a great misfortune.

CHRONIC DISORDERS:
THEIR SYMPTOMS AND CAUSES

In case of chronic pain, disorder, or trouble, there are very specific symptoms before the attack. If these symptoms are studied using the methods described earlier, you can use various healing practices to revert the pre-ailment symptoms, and save yourself from these pains, or aches, or other disorders. If you are successfully able to avoid a chronic disorder, the healing practices and allied precautions become so spontaneous, you will automatically remove the causing factors. Let's look at specific examples to see how this works in practice.

Chronic Pain

Chronic pain—migraine, sciatica, or any other such pain—attacks when there is an accumulation of fatigue so the general stamina of the body is low. An irregular lifestyle, a disturbance of the body functions (indigestion, constipation, excessive exertion, lack of appetite, etc.), exposure to cold, not enough sleep, stressful or noisy environments, are some of the factors that trigger chronic pain. For example, while recovering from a minor ailment like a cold, you are tired, but for some reason or another you have to stay up late. The next day, you feel even more tired, and in addition to that, you have a hectic day at work. By evening you are really exhausted. At this point, you may feel some pre-symptoms of your chronic pain. If you decide to postpone all your activities at this stage in order to get some rest, get some sleep, do the previously described healing practices, and develop a good relationship with the ailing part, you can successfully avoid the pain not yet come. If you learn to be "with yourself" and are able to communicate with the ailing part, you will notice the circumstances leading to the nagging, chronic pain.

It may seem that the pain attacks you all of a sudden, sometimes in the middle of the night (especially in the case of sciatica), but it is not like that. There are always pre-symptoms declaring the arrival of a chronic pain. You must learn to chase your chronic pain like an enemy, which it is. This enemy attacks you at a particular target repeatedly. Each time you combat the attack, but the enemy comes back again. Combating each attack costs you time and energy; therefore, you decide to adapt another strategy. You begin to do an area study in order to know the path your enemy will take. The next time, you try to obstruct your enemy on the way and combat the pain there. If you repeatedly defeat this nagging enemy, one day, he or your pain may leave the territory.

Chronic Sore Throats

You repeatedly feel an irritation and discomfort in your throat. From time to time, upon getting up in the morning, you feel like you have a sore throat, or you get frequent sore throats every couple of weeks. Each time, it persists for a few days. As in the example for chronic pain, find out very carefully, with great concentration, the circumstances leading to this event. It could be due to small incidents, like drinking and eating something that was too hot or too cold, or maybe you had cold drinks with hot food. It could be due to other factors, such as polluted or dusty air. You should always avoid drinking anything that is too cold. This is also a preventive and precautionary instruction for those who do not apparently suffer from chronic sore throats. The second principal measure against a chronic sore throat is the practice of yogic cleansing exercises for the throat, nose, and chest. The details of the yogic practices called *jalneti* and *jaldhauti* have been described previously. These two practices help clean the throat and nasal passages, and make the inner cell lining of this region resistant to various throat and nasal infections. *Jalneti* and *jaldhauti* are also beneficial to combat air pollution.

Stomach Problems

To cure recurring stomach problems, you will have to search within to find the fundamental factors causing the problem. As I said earlier, each person must eat according to his or her constitution.

Some people have very strong power of digestion and are capable of digesting large quantities of heavy food, whereas others are very sensitive and cannot eat heavy, fatty, and fried food. They often have stomach problems. If these frequently occurring problems are ignored, the consequences are serious, and they may end up with stomach ulcers. Another very common cause for stomach ailments is alcohol. People with a *pitta* constitution are more sensitive to alcohol than others. To drink alcohol on an empty stomach is more dangerous than to drink it with food or after meals. Stomach troubles may also be caused due to the side-effects of certain pain-relieving and anti-arthritic drugs. Posture defects or stressful circumstances may also result in stomach ailments. Sitting too much in a slightly bent posture, traveling long distances and sitting in odd positions often become the cause for upset stomach. Some people retract their abdominal muscles when they are stressed. This affects the stomach musculature and nerves, and leads to indigestion, acidity, and ulceration.

This description of some causes of stomach ailments is given to help you search for factors that may cause your own particular problems. A person with a strong constitution may end up ruining his or her health by following an unwholesome life style and regimen, and may bring the body to a point where its healing capacities are tremendously reduced. On the other hand, a person with a weak and delicate constitution may enjoy a relatively healthy, peaceful, and long life by taking appropriate care, curing and healing him- or herself at the onset of minor health problems, and by using various preventive methods for cure.

If you are aware of the causes of various problems, you can remove them, and heal the ailing part with your mental and spiritual strength. In the case of stomach problems, a light abdominal massage should be given before going to bed and after getting up. You should also send *prāṇaśakti* to this area and mentally address this vital part of your body. With these precautions, and by removing troublesome factors, you should be able to cure yourself and prevent the problems from recurring.

Sleep-related Disorders

These are a common health problem, particularly with people from technologically advanced societies. Sleep is essential. It rates with breathing and eating. Yet, millions of people suffer from sleep disorders which ultimately lead to other health problems in addition to fatigue. These disorders are generally maltreated or ignored. Instead of searching for the causes which lead to sleep-related problems, patients are generally put to sleep with sedatives (sleep-inducing medicines). An excessive use of sleeping drugs has done tremendous harm during recent years. People get dependent, and when they stop taking these drugs, they begin to suffer from depression. Recently, I learned that, in Germany, one in eight children is given sedatives in one form or another. Health ministries and other government bodies in the West are very strict about the use of any medication outside their norms. Āyurvedic medicines, which stand the testimony of thousands of years, are not allowed to be sold in Western countries. To get permission to market them, our medicine must be tested on rats and other laboratory animals, which costs millions of dollars, in addition to abusing the poor animals. It is ironic to observe that, despite all this fuss about safety measures concerning drugs, humanity suffers tremendously from the abusive side effects of "approved" medical drugs.

Sleep is a natural phenomenon essential to revitalize body and mind. It is that state when our minds are closed to external knowledge. When we are unable to sleep, it means that we are unable to disconnect ourselves from the external world. This can be due to many reasons. Let's look into some of these so that we can begin the "search within" in order to find out the causes which make the nights restless.

My experience of working with people having sleep problems reveals that sometimes the causes of sleep disorders are external and superficial. Some people suffer due to a noisy environment, too much talking before going to bed, or stuffy bedrooms. For example, a colleague in Paris constantly complained of sleeplessness, and told me that without a sleeping tablet, she remained awake the whole night. One day, I asked her to try some of my methods of pre-sleep atmosphere, certain yogic exercises, and other instructions to this effect. She told me that it was not possible for her to do all this due to her circumstances. Because of a lack of space, she and her husband slept in their family room. Her husband smoked a lot and watched television until late at night. As I said earlier, all of us have different constitutions. Her husband was not affected, at least immediately, by his deeds, but she suffered because of the loud and stuffy environment, and became a victim of insomnia. In such conditions, any methods of yoga or healing will not be able to help you. First of all, you need to help yourself by changing your home into a more natural, peaceful, and pleasant place, so you are able to revitalize your body with appropriate sleep.

Another important thing to understand is that your body is not a machine that you can switch on and off. The process of sleep is a slow transition from activity to non-activity and rest. Some people lead very hectic lives: they live in a state of hyperactivity and do not build a pre-sleep atmosphere for themselves. They are unable to close themselves from the outer world and suffer from sleep problems. Such is the case with managers, executives, or other people with hectic jobs, or with working mothers who have a double job. These people need to create a special pre-sleep atmosphere by not talking too much (or too loud) about an hour before going to bed, doing breathing exercises and *savāsana* (see below). You must carefully study the external factors that hinder sleep and try to eradicate them.

Using the yogic posture, *savāsana,* and learning some breathing exercises to help you detach from the external world are easy methods to attain peaceful sleep.

SAVĀSANA AND BREATHING EXERCISES

Savāsana (or the dead body posture) is a yogic posture that involves imitating a limp, lifeless corpse which has attained complete rest. Do not be frightened by the name of this posture. You are only imitating that restful state in order to have a peaceful state of mind, temporarily disconnected from the activities of the world. For making this posture, lie down on your back with your legs a little apart, and palms of your hands facing upward (figure 17 on page 122). Loosen yourself completely. Your hands, feet, legs, and arms should be completely relaxed and not stretched out in a tense way. Make sure your forehead does not have a frown, and that your neck and shoulders are relaxed. Your back should be completely at rest. Let yourself loose like a sleeping baby. You will observe that by doing all this, your body feels heavier and heavier. If you have successfully attained this state, then

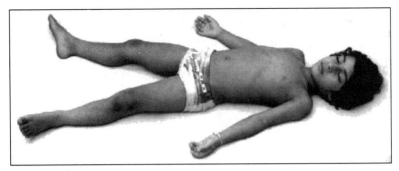

Figure 17. Śavāsana, or the dead body posture.

your breathing should automatically slow down. This latter happens because in a completely relaxed state, the body's requirement for oxygen lessens. You cannot attain this state of stillness until your mind is completely at rest. A state of fear caused by some noise or a bad dream can make you breathless even when you are lying down in your bed. Therefore, *śavāsana* is not merely lying down, but making yourself completely relaxed through the efforts of your mind. It is letting each part of your body relax and concentrating your mind on your body.

It is not always easy to make this posture. City dwellers are generally tense people, due to the hectic pace they live. For them, this āsana may be difficult to achieve, for, in the process of getting relaxed, they may get even more tense. When you are told to relax, you should just do it and not think about it. Relaxation is a state, and not something to rationalize through your thought process. Just do it.

Follow this simple method to facilitate the process of relaxation. Lie down as described above and bring your thought process to your body. Start thinking about your left foot. Think about the shape of your foot and its appearance. Then slowly come to your ankle and then to the leg. After you have reached the end of the left leg, begin the same way with the right foot, and finish this journey until the end of your right leg. Do this slowly, by getting familiar with each part of your body with the eyes of your mind. Similarly, begin with your left hand and go upward to your shoulder and follow it with the right side. Then bring your thought process to the central part of your body, from both front and back. After having done all this, "feel" your head and neck with your thoughts. This whole process will help you bring your mind from the outer to the inner, and a deep sleep will follow.

Breathing is necessary for survival. Modern biological sciences define breathing as a continuous interchange of gases between the organism and the external environment. The tissues of the body continuously consume oxygen and produce carbon dioxide. Breathing is a function. However, in the holistic system of Āyurveda, the phenomenon of breathing is looked upon from a different perspective. Breathing is a function but it is also our link to the cosmos. Air is one of the five fundamental elements which form the material reality of the universe. Entering the body, air is called *prāṇa*, or life. Without this cosmic link, we cannot exist. As soon as this link is broken, we are no more. When we are dead, all the five elements which constitute our physical being return to their cosmic pool. Various breathing practices involve the control of the vital air inside us, and are called *prāṇāyāma*. It will be necessary to learn some aspects of *prāṇāyāma* in order to get rid of sleep-related problems, as well as to learn to use other healing practices. The subtle details of *prāṇāyāma* are described a little later. Here, I will only introduce it so you can learn the initial part of healing.

To begin with, you should learn to follow your breath. "Following breath" means to break the mechanical process of breathing air in and out of your lungs. Instead of the air, you inhale *prāṇa*—life, itself. It carries the *prāṇaśakti* (the power of life). This power of life reaches each and every part of your body. You are alive because each and every part of your body is alive.

Returning to the subject of sleep, you should practice simple *prāṇāyāma* exercises each night, before going to bed. I suggest these also to people who do not suffer from sleep problems. This practice makes you calm, and provides the tranquil and peaceful sleep so vital to good health.

Sit down in a comfortable posture, preferably cross-legged. Keep your back straight but relaxed. Inhale slowly and profoundly. When the *prāṇa* (vital air) is inside you, close both your nostrils with your thumb and middle finger (figure 18 on page 124). Relax your back from the position of inhaling. After a few seconds, remove your fingers and let out the air slowly and steadily. Push all the air out. Once again, close your nostrils and hold the lungs without air for a brief interval. Then release the

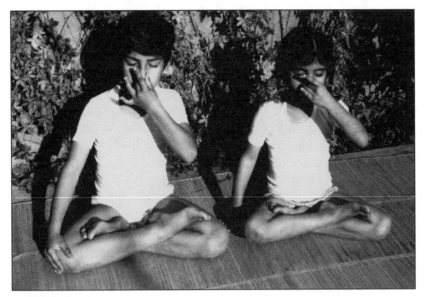

Figure 18. Prāṇāyāma.

nostrils and breathe deeply once again. Repeat this process about ten times each night before going to bed. To begin with, hold your lungs with and without air for a very brief period (a few seconds only). Gradually increase this interval, as well as the time taken to inhale and exhale the vital air. The process of inhaling and exhaling should be smooth and slow and not in jerks.

We will now move to the second part of the healing process, which involves evoking our inner subtle energy.

SUBTLE ENERGY AND THE ETERNAL SELF

According to yogic and Āyurvedic speculative thought, our material body contains a subtle body within it. We can call it the "energy corpse." This energy emanates from the main source of energy or the cause of our being—the self or *ātman*. In medical terminology, this self is named *jīva*. *Jīva* is indestructible, unchangeable, and eternal. It is the cause of consciousness, but it does not participate in the activities of the mind, body, and intellect. It is like a reflecting glass which sees all, but remains uninvolved. *Jīva* is a part of that eternal energy which is all-pervasive. Therefore, it is immense, as it belongs to the cosmic immensity. If we think that the material reality of our being, which is limited in space and time, is the only reality, then we cannot reach that eternal energy. At the time of death, it is this weightless, timeless, formless, and indestructible energy (or *jīva*) which separates from the physical body.

By realizing the true self and evoking the eternal within us, we are capable of opening an endless source of power for ourselves. It is this power which is responsible for the *yogasiddhis*.[5] It is this power which is named paranormal by some, and it is this power we are going to talk about in the context of healing. I am sure that many readers have heard about the great saints or yogis healing the sick with the touch of their hands.

In India, frequently a holy person gives you ashes from the fire of a sacred ceremony or some holy water for healing purposes. In Christianity, there is a great tradition of healing which continues from the founder of this religion, Jesus Christ. These traditions of healing, which are symbolic and subtle, were prevalent during the Middle Ages in Europe. However, in much of the Christian West, the ceremonies of healing have been completely forgotten with the advent of modern science, for science has treated traditional methods as mere superstitions. For the founding fathers of modern science, the body and the cosmos both function like a mechanical system. Thus, there is no place for soul (or *jīva*) and its eternal and immense power. This scientific system does not accept the evoked inner powers of a yogi or a saint, nor does it accept that there is tremendous capacity in each human being for establishing a link with eternal and immutable energy. Therefore, according to the Western way of thinking, there is neither a healer nor one to be healed.

However, despite the fundamental philosophy of the modern scientific and medical community, a large majority of us have had experiences which can be termed as mystical or paranormal. Some strong believers in the man-machine theory term these experiences products of hallucination or chance. In a traditional society like India, these phenomena are not considered paranormal. They are considered as normal, but it is realized that they

---

[5] For details of the *yogasiddhis*, see Part III of my book *Patañjali's Yoga Sūtras*.

fall beyond our sensory perception. Reality is not limited to the narrow framework of our sensual perception. What we perceive with our senses is only a part of the cosmic reality; it is not all of what is there. Our story of extra-sensory perception and its use in healing begins by learning to recognize our immutable eternal self so we can use this immense power to prevent illness and heal our destructible, vulnerable physical self. This whole discussion might sound very profoundly philosophical at this stage, but you will see that by following a three-step procedure with perseverance and concentration, it is possible for everyone to benefit from healing methods.

1. Learning breathing practices (or *prāṇāyāma*) and working with the subtle body;

2. Concentrating on *nābhi cakra*, or the navel point;

3. Concentrating on *hṛdya*, or the solar plexus.

BREATHING PRACTICES
AND THE SUBTLE BODY

Normally, many of us do not pay attention to our most vital activity—breathing. The process of inhaling and exhaling is a routine mechanical activity. Learn to break this mechanization. Stop reading this book for a moment, close your eyes, inhale deep by following the passage of the vital air inside you with your thoughts. When your lungs are full with this vital energy, hold the air in the lungs for a few seconds and then release the air very smoothly and slowly. When all the air is out, then think about the next breath and the volume of air you are going to take inside you again. Let it go inside your body very slowly and rhythmically. Let it stay inside you for a few moments of complete stillness. Then this vital air should be let out in the same slow and rhythmical fashion as was done for its inward journey.

To begin with, for two weeks, you may do this simple practice 5 to 10 times immediately after getting up and before going to bed. You may do this practice at any other time of the day except immediately after a meal when it is difficult to breathe deeply. It is essential to do these breathing exercises regularly. It takes about a minute to do these exercises in "aware breathing" in the morning before beginning your day and at night before ending your day. This activity will help you to break the mechanization in the process of breathing and will slowly make you realize that this process is your cosmic link; it is life, and it is energy.

After doing the above-described exercises for two weeks, make an effort to slowly increase the time of inhalation, holding the lungs full of air, exhaling, and holding the lungs without air. The passage of the vital air should be slow and smooth. The air should not enter or leave your body in a stop and go fashion or in jerks. After the intake of the vital air, close your nostrils with your thumb and middle finger (see figure 18 on page 124). Keep the air inside you as long as you comfortably can. While holding the air inside you, make sure that your body is not tense, and relax from the effort of inhaling. Slowly remove your fingers, and let the air out in a smooth and rhythmical fashion. When all the air is out, close your nostrils once again with your thumb and middle finger to hold the lungs without air for some time. Remove your fingers and inhale slowly and smoothly for the second round of this exercise.

To summarize, you have four steps to do: 1) slow, smooth, and profound intake of vital air; 2) closing the nasal passage, relaxing the body and holding the air inside; 3) letting the vital air out slowly and smoothly; 4) blocking the nasal passage again to hold the lungs without air.

Do this practice for about two weeks or until you feel self-confident. Do it regularly in the mornings and in the evenings. An irregular practice delays the progress in increasing the timing of the four steps described earlier.

During the next two weeks, do the same exercises, but not merely as a breathing exercise. While inhaling, think of the cosmic power your body is being provided. Let this power circulate throughout your body. Let all the blocked channels open so that the energy you are taking in can be well-distributed to each and every part of your body. The distribution of energy in the body takes place through the channels of the subtle body within the physical body. Concentrate while inhaling the vital air, and feel that this vital energy is being channeled to each part of your body. Let there be a free flow of energy. At the initial stages, during the process of inhalation, you may not be able to visualize the whole of your body all at once. Make an effort to channel the energy in different parts with each breath. Visualize the flow of energy in your arms, hands, and finger tips. Then let the energy flow in your head and subsequently to the other parts of your body. Pay special attention to those parts which have pain, are weak, or are vulnerable to ailments.

Once you have inhaled the vital air, close your nostrils, relax from the inhaling posture by loosening your back and shoulders, and feel the stillness inside you. During the process of exhaling, again visualize your subtle body and see the return of the cosmic element (air) which brought to you the goodness of life. After exhaling, close the nostrils again and think and feel nothing: just be. This is a momentary oneness with the cosmic energy of which all of us are a part.

If you are regular and spare only a few minutes daily for this practice, in six weeks time, you will be able to learn it perfectly well. What you are learning is not a magical wonder balm that you can apply on an ailing part to get instant relief. This practice helps you learn to recognize your inner reality, or the reality beyond your sensory perception. It helps you realize your cosmic link. From the Āyurvedic point of view, this practice helps to open blocked channels, and stops the accumulation of *kapha* in the body. When *kapha* blocks channels in the body, it blocks the passage of *vāta*. Those parts of the body where *vāta* is blocked do not get nourishment, and it is *vāta* which carries the products of *pitta* for the distribution in the body. In such circumstances, that particular part of the body begins to deform and a major disease is caused.

The above-described exercise should be done regularly and incorporated in your daily routine. Just as you brush your teeth every day, eat a few times a day, and consider sleeping essential, similarly, a few minutes should be spared daily to ensure the smooth and regular flow of energy in the body. This practice will slowly make you very sensitive to your body and enable you to detect the slightest disorder or ailment before it is expressed. You will also be able to find the reasons for any health problems that have no real symptoms, the ones you are hesitant to seek medical advice about. Our purpose here is not only to find the cause of the ailment but also the cure.

Do these practices regularly and increase the time from 2 minutes daily to 6 minutes—3 minutes in the morning and 3 minutes in the evening.

CONCENTRIC ENERGY POINTS OR *CAKRAS*

There are three principal channels of energy in the body, and from these three, the other channels branch out and spread throughout the body. These three main channels run from the lower part of the back to the middle of the forehead. They originate from left, right, and middle. The left channel is symbolized by the moon; the right by the sun. The sun and the moon channels cross each other and meet at the central channel six times (figure 19 on page 130). These meeting points are the *cakras* or energy circles. For a smooth flow of energy in the whole body, it is essential to purify these channels regularly.

The left (or moon) channel signifies inactivity, sleep, resistance. The right (or sun) channel is for motion, impetus, activities, movement, action, etc. The central channel represents the equilibrium between these two types of qualities.

For obtaining an equilibrium of the mind and the humors, a regular purification of the channels is essential in addition to adopting other features of the Āyurvedic way of life. For this purpose, I will describe some simple exercises in addition to the one you have already learned.

Begin with the breathing exercise (the last of the series) and do it for 4 to 5 breaths. Then do the same, but only with the right nostril. Close the left nostril with the thumb of the left hand (see figure 20 on page 130). Inhale through the right nostril slowly, smoothly, and deeply. Now close the right nostril with the ring finger of the same hand (figure 18, page 124). Relax your shoulder and back from the effort of inhaling. After a few seconds, lift your middle finger. The left nostril should be kept closed with the thumb of the right hand. After letting all the air out, close your right nostril, also using the middle finger again. Repeat this exercise 4–5 times with the right nostril. While doing so, concentrate on purifying the sun energy channel. Follow its passage downward and upward while inhaling and exhaling respectively. Do the same

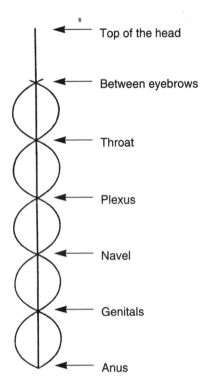

Top of the head

Between eyebrows

Throat

Plexus

Navel

Genitals

Anus

Figure 19. The three principal channels of the subtle body and their intersection correspond to six cakras.

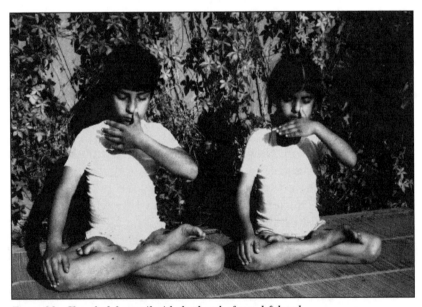

Figure 20. Close the left nostril with the thumb of your left hand.

with the left nostril while keeping the right nostril closed with the right thumb. Concentrate on the purification of the moon channel this time.

The next step of this practice is to alternate between left and right while doing the rest the same way. Inhale from the right nostril while keeping the left closed with your left thumb. Close also the left nostril, hold the breath for few seconds and exhale from the left nostril while using your ring finger to keep the right closed. After exhaling, close both nostrils again, and hold the lung without air for a few seconds. Now inhale from the left nostril and so on.

The first practice is done to purify the sun channel, and the second is done to purify the moon channel. The third practice is for creating a balance between the two, and for strengthening the central energy channel (balance). The same vital air is circulated from the left to the right, crossing all the energy *cakras*. This practice activates the dormant subtle energy.

Figure 21 (page 132) illustrates all three practices to make comprehension easy. The cross lines show closed nostrils, and arrows show the direction of the passage of the air. The circles with arrows show the movement of the vital air within the body.

I emphasize that you should do all the three practices daily for 2 to 3 minutes in the morning after getting up, and for the same amount of time before going to bed each night. The exercise should be used as a preventive measure to ward off small ailments. On the physical level, this cleans the respiratory tract and lungs. On a more subtle level, the exercise helps open the channels for a free flow of energy and helps you detect any minor, but not yet expressed, ailment. These practices revitalize the energy *cakras* and render a glow to one's complexion.

There are other benefits from these practices. We will now discuss their use for healing specific ailments. You need a complete mastery and concentration of the breathing practices to use them for healing ailments. After you have learned to heal yourself, you may use these practices for others. Use the following instructions to get started.

Sit in a relaxed posture and begin to concentrate on the ailing part. Converse with it as described earlier, and give it the assurance of a cure. Then, begin with your breathing practices. When you are inhaling the vital air, send all this vitality directly to the af-

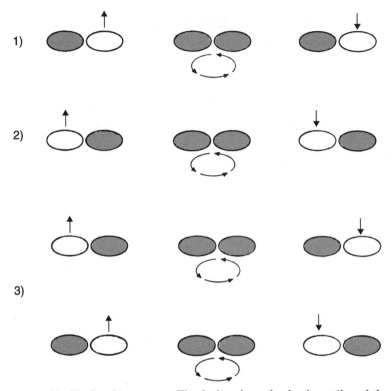

Figure 21. The breathing process. The shadow shows the closed nostril, and the arrows show inhalation and exhalation.

fected part. When you are holding the breath, let this vital energy circulate in the affected part, and irrigate that part with vitality. While exhaling, you are throwing out all that is blocking the flow of energy in the affected part. After that, when you are staying without air, it is the moment for assimilating energy in the weak and vulnerable part so that it rejuvenates and gets rid of the pain, tension, blockage, or whatever the case may be.

You require four qualities for healing: persistence, patience, perseverance, and concentration. You must realize that healing is the reversal of a process that gives rise to disharmony: mostly, a state of imbalance and disharmony has been left unattended at the initial stages. It takes some time until it becomes powerful enough to show its symptoms, and you call it an ailment. Therefore, the process of reversal from disharmony and imbalance to a state of equilibrium and health also requires some time. You are the conductor of your orchestra for all your physical and mental functions. A good conductor is able to detect a light fault of melody even in a big group. The players and their instruments are both checked and the orchestra rehearsal goes on until the melody is perfected. A healer needs similar qualities to a conductor.

Always be hopeful and tell yourself: "I am going to cure myself, I will cure myself, I am sure I can cure myself." Go on using the above-described methods as many times as you can, when and wherever possible. Just bring all your thoughts to the ailing part, give your love and care to it, and irrigate it with vital energy.

HEALING OTHERS

You cannot learn to heal others without practicing these methods on yourself. Healing others involves forming a connection with the other person. You may touch the affected part of the suffering person, or you may hold your hand at a little distance from it. Healing is also possible from a far away place, provided you know the exact details of the ailment and you are able to visualize it in detail.

You must be very careful in healing others and should always remember that you are forming only a channel between the vast Cosmic Energy and the suffering person. Do not concentrate on someone's ailment without forming your own link with the Cosmic Energy. If this is not done, in the process of healing others, you may end up taking their troubles and sufferings on you. That is why I emphasize again and again that you should learn to practice healing methods on yourself first, and attain success, before attempting to help others. You should learn that it is not the "I" of the worldly, mutable, and material body that is the healer. It is the indestructible, immutable, and eternal self of an individual (soul or *ātmā*) which has the power of healing (or *ātmaśakti*). Therefore, for healing, establish a link from the eternal within yourself to the eternal Cosmic Energy. Breathing practices are the first step for evoking *ātmaśakti*. I will discuss two more yogic concentration practices for evoking the dormant power of the Self and channeling that energy for healing.

For healing others, you must learn a higher level concentration practice, popularly known as meditation in the West. In this practice, you try to bring your mind to one concentric point of energy within your body. For the present purpose of healing, I have chosen the two energy points of the body: 1) *nābhi* or the navel point; and 2) *hṛdya*, popularly known as the solar plexus. The navel point is considered the central energy point of the physical body and its humors. It is said that by concentrating on this point, you can attain knowledge about your body functions.[6]

HEALING BY
CONCENTRATING ON THE BODY

Nābhi or the Navel Region

Sit in a comfortable posture, preferably cross-legged. Relax yourself using breathing practices previously learned. After your mind is still and free of the external thoughts, try to concentrate upon the navel point. Make sure your body is completely relaxed, and that your abdomen is not retracted. Shun all other thoughts from your mind and be persistent in bringing your mind to your navel point. When you are successful in achieving a state of stillness, and your mind has only one object—that is, your navel point— then begin to imagine the concentric circles of energy around this point (figure 22 on page 135). Slowly, the circles around this point will grow bigger and bigger, and will envelop your whole body. When you have achieved this state, and you find yourself within this envelope of energy, you will be in a state of stillness. Try to prolong this period by constant practice and persistence. Slowly, the concentric point of energy within, and the circles around, will become harmonious. These energy circles, seen at a state of stillness, are also called "aura" by some. Each one of you may see different forms and colors of this energy. This information will reveal the state of your humors.

If the humors are balanced and you are at peace with yourself, then you will "see" harmonious and still circles. If you have

---

[6] See *Patañjali's Yoga Sūtras*, Part III, sūtra 29.

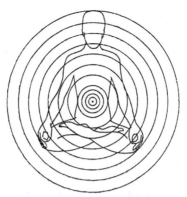

Figure 22. Visualize the concentric circles of energy around the navel point.

an excess of *vāta*, your energy circles will be vibrating, and you will have difficulty in prolonging the state of concentration, or the process of concentration may give you anxiety.

Various shades of red, orange, and blue in your energy fields are indicative of *pitta* domination. If these colors are too strong, they speak of a vitiated *pitta*. That means that there is an excess of heat in your body. You tend to suffer from problems related to digestion.

White, thick, opaque, and viscous layers in your energy circles indicate the domination of *kapha*, and the constricted passage of energy in the body. It also indicates restraint and a lack of ease of self-expression. This practice will help you analyze yourself in the Āyurvedic way.

For healing a particular disorder after having "visualized" the energy envelope around you, concentrate your thoughts on the affected part. By doing so, you channel the energy in this part. This way of healing is of a higher order than the methods described previously. Here, you are going beyond language and words. You are opening your inner vision. You are in a higher realm of energy and merely by concentrating on the affected part, you are revitalizing and curing it.

Earlier we discussed talking to the affected part of your body. You have also learned to control the vital breath and to channel this energy to the affected and weak parts of your body. Now, you are dealing with a higher level of communication, where you are supplying the suffering organism with life-giving force, helping it to harmonize with the rest. It is difficult to explain all this in words, as it is beyond words.

These spiritual methods of healing cannot be learned or practiced at the time of need. You need persistent training to arrive at a higher level of consciousness. Only then is it possible to develop the capacity to shut yourselves completely from the external sensual world to be one with the inner eternal energy. You should do these concentration practices every day for a few minutes, and slowly you will make progress in achieving a state of stillness. This will help you find your balance, and you will get to know yourself. You will become very sensitive to your body and able to foresee the illness not yet come. Thus, this practice will help you prevent ailments at a very elementary stage, and will guide you to avoid health-damaging behavior. However, in the case of a more advanced or chronic ailment, you will need to do this practice for a longer time than just a few minutes daily.

To apply this practice on others, you must concentrate on the person concerned and then bring your thoughts specifically to his or her navel point. However, doing this practice on others involves a still higher level of concentration than doing it on yourself. In the former case, you have to transcend yourself completely and enter into the other person's energy field.

THE *HṚDYA,* OR SOLAR PLEXUS

In yoga and Āyurveda, this area is considered the site of *ātmā,* or soul, or the Self. As you know, it is this light which holds our body together. It is *that* which is the cause of consciousness, and it is our real, immutable, eternal Self. Thus, *hṛdya* is where the soul resides (if we may use this word "reside," as soul does not have any substance). It is not easy to concentrate on something which is non-sensuous (beyond the scope of senses). It takes time and effort to transcend sensual reality. Therefore, begin to concentrate on some symbolic representation of the eternal energy: it may be a flame, the sun, or the syllable "OM" (figure 23 on page 137), or any other symbol you prefer. It is better to select a neutral symbol that has no association or involvement, as otherwise your thoughts may wander elsewhere. When the con-

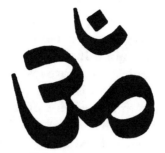

Figure 23. OM.

centration is uninterrupted on the symbol located in the solar plexus, you are slowly enveloped in an aura of energy, and will find yourself sublimated in this energy.

Repeat this exercise every day for a few minutes. The first stage of success should be the uninterrupted concentration on your chosen symbol at the solar plexus. The next stage of concentration is that you are not thinking about your symbol or visualizing it. It is just there as an image on your mind. Rationality and language are lost. You and this symbol submerge into each other and become one. The final stage is when the identity of the symbol is also lost, and your entire being is sublimated in Cosmic Energy.

The higher levels of concentration are difficult to achieve, and you may face hurdles, like fearfulness, sweating, or trembling. With regular practice and perseverance, these hurdles are removed. When your mind becomes steady, and you are able to concentrate on the symbol which is the cause of your being, and which is a part of the eternal Cosmic Energy within you, then you will be able to heal.

Visualize the weak and affected part and concentrate on it. It is just an inner visualization, and not seeing with the sense of sight. The next step is to concentrate on the solar plexus region (described earlier) and sublimate yourself with the eternal energy. This way, you submerge your physical being, along with the ailment, in the eternal Cosmic Energy. The limitless Cosmic Energy is very strong. It opens all the blocked channels and helps bring the body's humors in balance. However, you should remember that to evoke this eternal energy, you have to go beyond sensuous reality, and it is not all that easy! It is a long and hard path. Once the goal is achieved, you should not think that this achievement will stay with you permanently. You need to regularly practice controlling your mind. If you discontinue your concentration practices, your achievements are lost. The mind's basic nature is to wander. But the mind is only controlled by the mind, itself. You have to learn to apply reins on the activities of your mind by directing your thought process to a desired point.

You cannot begin to learn healing practices when you are already weak and sick. At this stage, both your mental and physical capacity are reduced. Therefore, you should learn the practices that lead to healing when you are healthy and energetic. You will realize that by doing so, you are not only able to maintain good health, but you also have another view of the universal reality. Your horizons will expand. Your physical and mental power will increase, and you will develop the intuitive and spiritual powers often termed as "paranormal" in the West. You will be able to foresee many events related to you and others close to you. You will develop the mental power to influence others. This, however, should not be used to achieve negative goals, like stealing or influencing others to achieve your selfish motives, or for cursing others. This will bring you back negative energy in one form or another. You should use your inner strength only for good.

People who wish to heal others, or who want to become professional healers, should practice concentration for a long time. They should remain humble and never entertain the feeling of arrogance. They should continue their daily concentration practice to learn more. In my opinion, healers should have a thorough knowledge of the holistic medical system. In other words, they should not exclusively use psychological and spiritual therapeutic measures while ignoring rational therapy. Healers can also work in cooperation with good physicians who provide appropriate rational therapeutic measures.

HEALING WITH NATURAL FORCES

Ethnic medical practices from all over the world include healing rituals, prayers, or other ceremonies associated with certain holy places, rivers, stones, mountains, trees, or with some specific astronomical time. In the ancient medical literature of Āyurveda, healing rituals are largely based upon the worship of the five fundamental elements that constitute our material reality. Out of the five basic elements particularly worshipped for healing purposes were air, fire, and water. As you know, these three are directly related to the three humors. Out of these three elements, fire was perhaps worshipped the most in ritualistic and sacrificial traditions. Rivers, lakes, and ponds are sacred for water worship. The god of wind is worshipped, and there are many references to this in the Vedic literature. The worship of earth is more common for showing gratitude for giving food, shelter, and medicines rather than for healing. There is a tradition of worshipping certain trees for healing, for their medicinal properties, and to show gratitude for their healing capacities.

Nature's power is infinite. A tiny seed hides in it an enigma, for when it gets appropriate earth, water, light, air, and space, it flourishes and grows into a mighty tree in time. It does not need a laboratory, library, or the human thought process. It lives in harmony with nature. A tree symbolically represents the whole cosmos made up of the five elements. By establishing a harmonious relationship and friendship with a tree, we build our cosmic connection. By worshipping the five elements, we connect ourselves to the natural powers.

When a sick person goes to a sacred and holy place, whether it is Varanasi in India, or Lourdes in France, or Mecca in Saudi Arabia, or makes any other such pilgrimage (figure 24 on page 140), it is with a strong wish and faith that the power of the holy place will cure him or her. With this process, the person's inner power is evoked. The helplessness and hopelessness which is caused by the ailment slowly vanishes with the rise of his or her inner power (or ātmaśakti). Similarly, a holy place is holy because it has this power from the prayers and faith of millions of people for thousands of years. We purify a place with our thoughts, will, and with good deeds of friendship, compassion, and generosity.

Establishing a connection with the five elements, and showing gratitude toward them, evokes your inner consciousness, and widens your vision of reality. Under a beautiful blue sky, in an open space, try to assimilate the energy from vastness and expansion (figure 25 on page 140). Concentrate your thoughts on expanding your inner self with this vastness.

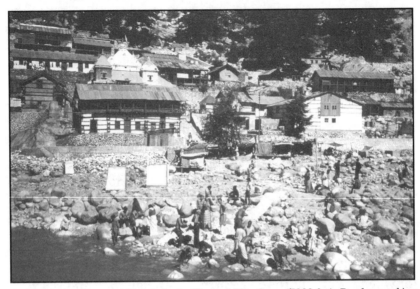

Figure 24. The Gangotri Temple in the Gharwal Himalayas (7000 feet). People are taking healing baths.

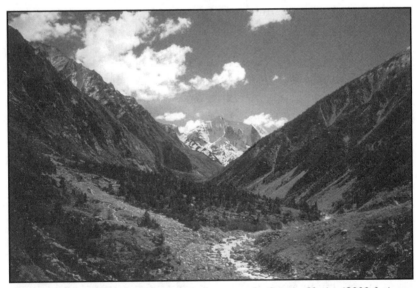

Figure 25. In the high Himalaya mountains, near the Ganges Glacier (9000 feet), one can experience ākasla, or ether.

I have already described several breathing practices for experiencing our vital cosmic connection through this activity. Both ether and air give rise to *vāta* in your body. Air, in normal conditions, is life-giving. When it is vitiated, it is destructive. It uproots trees, destroys houses, causes high tides, etc. Similarly, *vāta* (derived from ether and air) performs its functions well in a state of equilibrium, but when vitiated, it causes havoc in the body. Besides maintaining balance with nutrition and medicine, some healing practices based on *Athārvaveda* can be used as a preventive and curative for *vāta* disorders. These healing methods include concentrating and praying to the two elements which form *vāta*.

While doing the breathing practices described earlier, concentrate on the vastness of space (ether). When your mind attains stillness, then repeat the following:

> Oh ether! Oh air! I bow to your magnanimity and generosity. Please be kind to me. Please keep *vāta* in balance in my body. May *vāta*, which is derived from both of you, perform well its functions in my body. May it provide me with courage and fearlessness. Like both of you, which are all-pervasive and all-nourishing, let *vāta* nourish each and every part of my body. Oh, powerful ether and air, grant me harmony. May good sense prevail in me, and may I avoid doing all which vitiates *vāta*. I have this humor in harmony. Let me be free from the disorders created by *vāta*. Oh, mighty ether and air, remain in your natural order in this cosmos, as well as within me. I know your virtues and merits. I know that you are responsible for my body movements and mind activities. It is you who nourish my whole body with nutrients by circulating blood everywhere with your virtue. I survive by taking in and out the vital air from your vast stores. It is your power which helps me get rid of poisons from my body. You put words into my mouth and are responsible for feeling, sensation, etc. My natural urges are guided by you, and the result of one such urge is procreation. It is you who helped in my formation when I was in my mother's womb. Oh wind, and ether, bless me so that all the *vāta* functions are well-performed in my body. Let *vāta* not vitiate in my old age. Give me sense so that I eat according to place and time to keep *vāta* in order. May I live long without *vāta* ailments which tend to increase during old age. Oh wind and ether, bless me for harmony and equilibrium of *vāta*. I bow to your might. Let harmony prevail!

I have given you a general text, but you may change it according to your needs. For example, you know that *vāta* is responsible for the formation of the fetus. If you are expecting a baby, then concentrate on ether and wind every day, and pray for the right formation of your baby. Think about the details of the formation of your baby, its growth and development.

> Oh wind and ether, I bow to your might. I pray to you for the harmony of *vāta* in my little one. I know that you are responsible for its growth and formation. I pray to you for the formation of well-developed and well-formed organs in my baby. Oh ether and wind, let my baby be well-formed and beautiful. Let my baby have all healthy and complete organs in the right proportions. Oh wind and ether, I pray to you for the well-being of my baby.

You may add more to this text, abiding by all the functions of *vāta*.

If you feel that all the other functions of *vāta* are all right in you, but you lack courage and strength, then you may pray specifically for these two qualities to the formative elements of *vāta*.

> Oh ether and air, you are very bold and life-giving. Oh wind, you are very strong. You give *prāṇa* (life) to all living beings. Your constant movements provide a refreshing feeling to all the living creatures. You help the growth of seeds. Oh ether, it is your vastness which gives us space to be here in this universe. Both of you are responsible for all the *vāta* functions in me. I pray for harmony in this humor. Bless me with courage and strength. You have blessed me with physical and mental activities. I breathe well and my blood circulates well, nourishing all parts of my body. I hear, feel, and speak. I am grateful to you for all that. But I lack courage and strength. I want to be bold, strong, and courageous. For that, I seek your blessings. Oh wind and ether, I am very well aware of your generosity. I know that you will not disappoint me. I pray to you to give me courage and strength. Please give me courage and strength. Let me have courage and strength that I can use for my own benefit, and for the benefit of others. Give me courage to get rid of my timid behavior. Give me strength so I am able to express myself well. Oh ether and air, I pray to you to bless me so that I become courageous and strong. With this wish, I bow to your might!

For other signs of vitiated *vāta*, you may prepare for yourself similar kinds of texts.

The inspiration for these healing methods comes from *The Athārvaveda*, which prescribes healing mantras along with specific ceremonies. You may call the text presented here a mantra or a healing method. You can use this healing method for yourself as well as for healing others. For others, let the suffering person lie down, relax, and breathe deeply. Then you can start to read the prepared text loudly. In the healing text, the power of the elements giving rise to humors should be acknowledged, gratified, and repeatedly requested to reestablish harmony and to cure ailments which concern that particular humor.

For the healing practices of *pitta*, we address to the sun or the fire, which are the sources of heat and light. The ceremony addressed to the sun is done by facing toward the sun. Do not look directly at it, as it is harmful for the eyes. Look at the sun through leaves and trees, or just concentrate on its image by closing your eyes. Ceremonies addressed to fire are usually done by proper sacrificial rituals. Symbolically, you may also concentrate on a flame, but do not stare at it, as it is harmful for the eyes. Just look at the flame and then concentrate on its image with closed eyes. Repeat the following healing mantras.

> Oh sun, I bow to your power which gives us life through your light and heat. You provide me with the capacity to see with my eyes. Your light shows me the beautiful universe of color and form. Inside my body, you are *pitta*—the fire of life. It is you who provide heat in my body, who give me hunger and thirst, and because of your grace my body has fire *(agni)* to digest the food I eat. You are generous, you provide me with softness and luster. Your light and heat make me cheerful. It is with your kindness that I assimilate knowledge. You provide me intellect. Oh mighty sun, I thank you for your kindness and generosity. I pray to you to regulate *pitta* in my body. I pray to you to save me from all kinds of fevers which are caused by vitiation of *pitta*. Bless me, Oh mighty sun, so that I do not suffer from the vitiated *pitta*. May the fire within me be regulated. I may feel hungry and thirsty according to my requirements, but I may not consume more than my need. Save me from too much heat in my body, which causes skin eruptions. Let there be balance in my life. Let good sense prevail in me so that I do not do anything to vitiate *pitta*. I am satisfied and contented with whatever I have. Bless me with patience and endurance. Save me from anger. Oh ever-generous sun, with your abundant light, enlighten me so that I can see the real light within me. I pray to you, oh brilliant sun, to sharpen my intellect. Oh sun, I bow to you. Bless me with balance and harmony.

As I have described earlier for *vāta*, for *pitta* also, you may make your diverse texts for getting rid of specific disorders, or for enhancing certain capabilities. For example, people who are engaged in intellectual and creative work may make prayers for increasing their power, intellect, and creativity. People who have problems with vision may also do these healing practices.

The idea here is not to give you something ready-made, but to teach you the fundamental basis of healing. After having learned this, you may elaborate these methods according to your own need, place, and time. But you should not forget that these healing methods are not exclusive of other Āyurvedic health care practices. They say that God helps those who help themselves. You may call the forces of nature as gods (as the Hindus do, or as the ancient Greeks and Egyptians did), or you may not. But the fact of the matter is that these energies are very powerful, and are beyond human control. If you do everything to vitiate a particular humor, and then try healing practices to get rid of ailments caused by this vitiation, your work may not be productive.

For example, if someone has a problem with skin eruptions or herpes, he or she is evidently suffering from *pitta* vitiation. If this person does not make an effort to appease his or her vitiated humor, is careless and does things to further vitiate this more, evidently, the suffering will increase. This person's efforts to cure his or her ailment through healing will be futile. It is as if you have a fire somewhere, and with one hand, you go on adding fuel to it, and with the other hand, you use a fire extinguisher to put this fire out. Would this not be a ridiculous action?

For preventing and curing *kapha*-related disorders, you should seek the blessings of Mother Earth and water. Concentrate upon these two elements by performing a small ceremony, just as we did earlier with breathing practice and looking at the sun or a flame. To show your gratitude to earth and water, you may sit beside a natural source of water, like a river, lake, or sea. Bow to this water source and earth.

Oh Mother Earth, from you all creatures are born, and after death, they go back to you. You are large-hearted and caring. You provide firmness to the trees. You provide a womb for the seeds. You give us millions of things for our well-being and comfort. Oh Mother Earth, you are varied, vast, and generous. You symbolize fertility, and thus continuity for us. You have an integral relationship with water. You hide water in your womb. Your ponds, lakes, and rivers provide us with life-giving water. Even your deserts hide oases somewhere. You have vast seas and oceans. You give shelter to millions of living beings. Oh Mother Earth, you and water, in the form of *kapha*, provide structure and form to my body. It is you who make bones, muscles, and other parts of my body. Just as you provide us with body structure, you also give us all the materials which give structure to our houses. Oh Mother Earth, I am grateful to you for your care, protection, and generosity, and I bow to you. Bless me so that *kapha* in my body remains in equilibrium. Bless me so that a good sense prevails in me which leads me to do all to keep *kapha* in equilibrium. Bless me so that I remain free from greed. Give me strength and forbearance. Save me from being lazy. Bless me for the harmony of *kapha* in my body. Let *kapha* accumulate nowhere, as its accumulation will block the passage of *vāta*. Oh earth and water, save me from weariness and lassitude. May *kapha* in my body stay in balance. I bow to your generosity and love. You give me structure and form. You provide me hands to work with and feet to walk on. I express to you my gratitude and seek your blessings. I pray to you for harmony and balance.

As I have said for the other two humors, here, too, you may make your own text for healing specific *kapha*-related disorders. For example, you know that *kapha* is responsible for potency and hence fertility. If you are desiring progeny, you may practice these methods and seek blessings for increasing your potency and hence progeny. Similarly, if you sleep a lot, and tend to feel depressed easily, you may write another prayer directed to earth and water for curing your specific problems.

OTHER HEALING METHODS

After having talked about healing practices related to the three humors and five elements, let us now come to other diverse methods of healing. These healing methods are mostly based upon faith in something. It may be a temple, a pilgrimage center, a holy tree, a holy mountain, a holy stone, a holy person, a sacred building, or anything of reverence. It may also be a pledge, like that of fasting. Such healing practices are used all over India in folklore medicine. They are, in fact, not exclusively used for healing, but for making any wish. For example, a temple, or an old peepal (figure 26 on page 146) or banyan tree are all considered holy in India. Someone may make a wish like, "May all go well with my acting in the play which we are performing in the open air. May there be no rain on the day of performance. If my wish is ac-

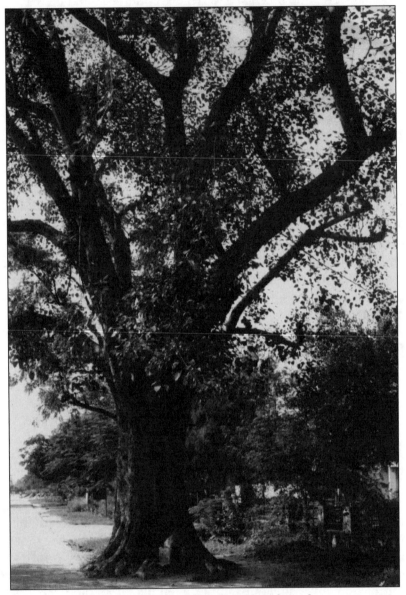

Figure 26. The healing peepal tree and the little temple underneath.

corded, I will come and light here five oil lamps." Or, "May my husband or wife stop smoking. Oh mighty banyan tree, accord me my wish. If my wish is granted, I will come and light a lamp each day for fifteen days." In a temple, offerings may be involved when the wish is granted. A pledge of austerity may involve some kind of fasting. Similarly, one may pledge to travel to a holy place if a wish is granted. For example, if someone has trouble with his or her feet and legs, this person may pray to the far away temples in the Himalayas and say, "Oh Great Lord of the Mountains (Siva), if my ailment is cured and my legs are again healthy, I will visit your holy abode." Most of these temples in the mountains involve a lot of walking (figure 27 on page 148). Therefore, such a wish has a significance of walking.

I have discussed this to convey to you that you might find your holy tree, or a holy stone, or your favorite Seine, Danube, Thames, Rhine, or Ganges, a peaceful mountain, a special corner of the forest, or an old rock in your own surroundings. By concentrating your thoughts on this particular object, you are evoking your own inner energy, which helps to heal you. By establishing harmony within yourself and with your surroundings, everything is possible. You should try to establish a good relationship and respect for all living and non-living things around you. They may be the four walls of your apartment, your car, a cherry or mango tree growing in your yard. You will see that by doing so, you will achieve *shanti* (peace and harmony) and good health. It is only with good health that you can look forward to material gain and spiritual achievement. Do not postpone your health problems and do not let your ailments get the best of you. When an ailment is at an irreversible state, these health care methods will not work. Health is like a fragile piece of porcelain; if it is not caught before hitting the ground, it breaks into pieces. Therefore, the time to act is now.

Some other simple methods of healing that are generally used as home remedies consist of exorcizing the ailment through a medium like a leaf, flower, or a piece of wood. This object acts as a medium between the sick and the healer. This simple practice is often taught to small children, who are generally very sincere in their efforts. Reality has a much wider dimension for them than for most adults.

Let the patient lie down in a relaxed posture. Take a leaf or a flower in your hand. Concentrate on the affected part. Let us try

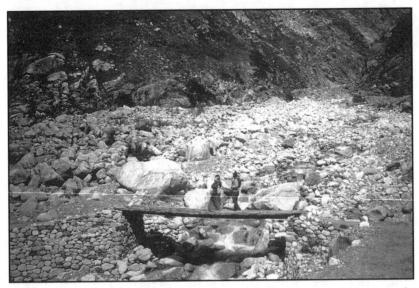

Figure 27. Fufilling the promise after being healed from an ailment. Trekking up to the Ganges Glacier.

to cure the headache. Stroke the head gently with the leaf or flower (see figure on page 105) and repeat the following:

> Oh pain, do not trouble this person. Leave his or her body. Withdraw from this person and enter into this leaf. Leave this person free. Do not make this person suffer with your presence. Just leave and enter into this leaf. I request you to leave this person and never to come back. You can enter into this leaf and travel to a far away lonely desert. Leave this person free from suffering. I request that you enter into this leaf.

Repeat this several times while stroking gently the head and forehead of the ailing person with the leaf. After the ceremony is over, take the leaf away and throw it in the garbage, or in a far away place, and say something like this:

> Let this energy be destroyed and disintegrated. It is not helping anyone. Oh leaf, I thank you for your help in extracting the negative energy from the ailing person and letting him or her be free of pain. I thank you for your help and goodness. I request you to destroy this pain completely so that it never comes back again.

HEALING THE MIND

Until now, we have discussed physical ailments and have not talked very much about the activities of the mind. It is essential that we are aware of the negative activities of the mind, so we can learn to curb them. They pollute both body and mind, and give rise to a number of physical and mental ailments. Āyurveda has used an ancient tradition (since the time of the *Athārvaveda*) to use healing ceremonies to get rid of the negative attributes of the mind. I cite below some mantras that were chanted by priests during these healing rituals.

> You, the man full of jealousy, extremely possessive about your woman, I pacify your jealous activities and detach you from anger and grief. As the earth is peaceful and does not entertain jealousy, just like that, your mind may not be the site for entertaining jealousy. Oh man, I let the anger related to your woman partner out from your heart just like an air blower throws out the air."[7]

In Āyurveda, there are four inner enemies which lead to dissatisfaction. We must continuously keep control of our mental activities and heal our damaged minds immediately from the effects of these negative qualities. If we do not pay attention to the damage caused by these negativities, we not only create mental disorders, but we may also become prey to a serious malady, like cancer. If we learn about these enemies of our health, we can avoid falling into their trap. The four principal enemies are desire, anger, attachment, and greed.

Desire

Desire, or *kāma*, is translated as sexual desire by some. It also means worldly pleasure, and the desire to possess various objects to that effect. It indicates possessiveness toward the people one loves. Desire (*kāma*) includes a longing for more and more sensuous pleasures, such as eating too much, seeing, talking, or listening indiscriminately, and an insatiable desire for sex. The desire

---

[7] *Athārvaveda*, VI, 18.

arises from dissatisfaction, and dissatisfaction gives rise to further desire.

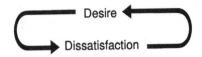

The world of desire is very enchanting, and our minds are attracted to it like magnets to iron. Wisdom lies in controlling the mind. An excess of desire—for things, people, sensuous pleasure—and a lack of self-discipline (or self-control) lead to eventual health problems. For example, excessive smoking, too much alcohol, too much sugar, etc., leads to trouble. People have plenty of excuses to cover up for their lack of self-discipline. They say they are smoking or drinking too much because they have some problems in their lives. Problems are not solved by creating new problems. The real solution to problems is to realize the impermanence of worldly pleasures and possessions, and making an effort not to hanker after them. It is essential to curb longings and cravings. Always remember that this dynamic universe is constantly changing; nothing stays forever in any place or with anyone. Even if we get something or somebody we are longing for, it does not put an end to our desires. One desire gives rise to another, and unfulfilled desires give rise to pain, anger, and frustration. They pave the way for both physical and mental ailments. A lack of self-control and excessive desires that give rise to dissatisfaction are particularly prevalent in our modern times because there is an obvious dearth of philosophical and religious training. It is essential to learn to control desire. To illustrate this, I will tell you the story of an old woman we heard about when we were children.

There was an old woman who lived in a hut in the forest. She was far away from town and there were no houses near her little hut. The old woman used to grow vegetables and grain crops for herself, and the forest was full of various kinds of fruits. The old woman had also planted some of her own fruit trees. Sometimes traveling merchants stopped and stayed the night at her place when it was too late to cross the forest. These merchants used to thank the old woman for her hospitality, and they gave her little presents. The old woman was happy and content. She was very busy with her plants, trees, and crops; she loved her surroundings. Many friendly birds and animals of the forests often visited her.

One day, some men came to the forest on their horses. They inspected the forest close to the old woman's hut. Some deal was made, and after a few days they started constructing a house not far from the woman's hut. Soon, a beautiful house with stone and wood was made. Some people came to live in this house. They used to go to town in their wagons and buy all kinds of comfort and luxury. The old woman, who was once content and happy suddenly became envious and filled with a desire to have her own beautiful house and all kinds of comforts. She prayed to the lord architect *Viśvakarmā* to be kind to her and get her a beautiful stone house like that of her neighbors. Due to the good *karma* of the old woman, lord *Viśvakarmā* granted her wish. The next morning, the old woman woke up in absolute delight, for she found herself in a big and beautiful house instead of her hut. The old woman looked in the corners of her new house and felt that it was big and beautiful, but empty. She had the desire to decorate it with beautiful furniture and things. For that she needed money. She prayed to the goddess of wealth *Lakśmī* to obtain some money. Again, because of the good past *karma* of the woman, she was blessed with some wealth.

With this wealth, she bought herself a horse and wagon, and went to town shopping for her house. There was such a variety of goods in town that the old woman was confused about what to buy. She looked in the shops for several days and at last bought the desired goods for her house. She kept so busy decorating the house that she forgot about her plants and trees who provided her food. When the house was decorated, she felt that she could not clean it by herself as it was too big. She also felt that she was a rich lady and it did not behove her to have a broom in her hand. She desired to have servants work for her. But she had already spent all her money. She prayed again, this time to the lord of lords, *Śiva*, to provide her with servants who will work for her. Again, on the grounds of her past good *karma*, the lord granted her wish. The servants started to do all her work. Good food and drinks were prepared for her. She got involved with her house and wealth, and slowly lost contact with the friendly animals and birds. She did not look after her plants, as the servants did all that for her. Eating and sleeping made the old woman fat and sluggish. She began to feel lazy and tired, and started having pains and swellings in different parts of her body. She wanted to have good health again.

She prayed to the sage of health, *Agniveśa*, this time. The sage appeared, and the old woman begged to him, "Oh wise one, with the blessings and boons of all the gods I am wealthy and comfortable. All I need is good health to enjoy all my possessions. I beg to you, Oh great sage of health, to make me healthy once again." The sage replied, "Listen to me, my lady, the stock of your good *karma* is over. I cannot help you. You have all and you want more. You must work for it in terms of good deeds." After saying this, the sage disappeared. The old woman had nostalgia for the old days when she used to go for long walks in the forest and collect fruits. She looked at her fat and ugly legs and her swollen feet. She realized that all this misfortune resulted from her desire to have a house like her neighbor's. In this process, she lost the greatest of her wealth—good health. Her peace and contentment was gone and she was regretting her past. She had once advised the merchants who passed that way to be content and satisfied with whatever they had, as desire was the root of all evil and unhappiness.

In order to learn self-control, we need to constantly remind ourselves about the bad effects of excessive desire and the importance of *santoṣa*. *Santoṣa* means "to be satisfied with whatever we have," so that we do not crave for things and people. It means that we obtain a stable mental state where we are not overwhelmed about "wants," and do not feel pained upon losing objects of comfort, the people we love, or any other sensuous pleasure. It means that we do not grieve over what is not there, and not get excited about what is there. It means that we are always thankful for whatever we have.

Anger

The second enemy of health is anger, or *krodha*. A state of anger makes you crazy, and leads to making wrong decisions. Anger destroys memory, raises the blood pressure, and affects the digestive system. You should always try to get rid of anger and find other ways to solve problems. If you think it is necessary to get angry in certain situations in life, then keep it to its theatrical role. Think always of the ridiculous part of anger. During moments of anger, try to detach *yourself* and look at yourself from another person's point of view. Perhaps you can begin to realize that anger is wasting emotions in a futile way. The same energy can be used for a better purpose.

If you tend to get easily irritated and angry, think also of getting your blood sugar, blood pressure, and digestion checked. Also make sure to get enough sleep. Anger is often related to desire. Unfulfilled desires and a state of dissatisfaction give rise to anger and irritation. Therefore, while dealing with enemy Number Two, we must keep in mind the enemy Number One.

Attachment

The third enemy of human health is attachment, or *moha*. Having too much attachment for a car, house, husband, wife, or children gives rise to anxiety and pain. Anxiety gives rise to imbalances in the body, makes us look old, causes our hair to turn gray and fall out, brings wrinkles and digestive problems. Anxiety may also give rise to arteriosclerosis (hardening of the arteries), hemorrhoids (piles), stomach ulcers, intestinal problems, and a number of other ailments.

We must learn to detach from "things" as well as from loved ones. Nothing stays for ever. The person we love so much may die, or may not love us. The house we are so fond of may be destroyed in a matter of seconds with an earthquake. All this may sound cruel, but these are the hard facts of life, and for keeping a healthy mind and body, we have to remind ourselves constantly of these eventualities. We need to make an effort to develop detachment from the objects and the people around us. This, however, does not mean that we should become pessimistic about life, or see only negative aspects. On the contrary, we should be optimistic, think that all will go well, and enjoy each moment! It is a privilege to be alive. Nevertheless, we can not ignore the fact that in this ever-changing, dynamic universe, anything can happen at any time. We need to prepare ourselves for all eventualities in order to avoid the pain not yet come.

Greed

The fourth enemy is greed, or *lobha*. People want more and more, and use all sorts of means to get it. An insatiable desire to have more and more is *lobha*. A bigger car, a bigger house, a country house, more money, more comforts—it makes a never-ending list. People overwork, live in stress and tension, ruin their present in hope of a better future, all because of *lobha*. In this process, they become victims of a great many serious diseases, such as hypertension, heart problems, many kinds of aches and pains, and they suffer constantly. They do not realize that the pleasures of living are worthless if life, itself, is endangered. Āyurveda ascertains that the first priority of life is life, itself. If you lose your health, fall prey to serious ailments, or die at an early age, all the possessions in the world are meaningless. Therefore, one of the most important things to have is *santoṣa* (satisfaction and contentment). This is possible when we learn to curb desire, anger, attachment, and greed. Most of the diseases of our times originate from stress and tension, which in turn are the products of the four negative attributes of the mind.

◊   ◊   ◊

Getting rid of desire, anger, attachment, greed, and attaining a mental state of *santoṣa* are important to avoid illness. It is also essential to develop a peaceful mental state in order to enhance our intuitive capabilities. To develop a power of "seeing more" than with sensory perception is essential for using previously described healing methods. Now, the question arises as to how we should proceed. Like any other learning, it is possible to imbibe the positive qualities and get rid of negative ones by constant effort and perseverance. We must not brush aside our actions; we must look at them introspectively. Then we can learn about the negative attributes of our mental activity and related social behavior. We need to be strict in order to teach ourselves mental discipline, and we learn just as small children learn to clean their teeth and other good habits. If we are interested in learning new things and values, if we are persistent, we can find time to think about the day's activities introspectively. We can correct ourselves whenever we feel that the mind was overpowered by one or more of these four enemies. Like this, slowly, we can learn the greatest of human qualities—*santoṣa*. This will lead to peace and harmony, and as you have already learned, harmony is the fundamental basis for health.

You may use the previously described methods of healing to get rid of the desire, anger, etc. The *Athārvaveda* provides many mantras, and I present another to help you devise your own text according to time and need.

Oh desire for physical pleasure, Oh desire for wealth, you are the cause of dispute between men and women. With your effect, a woman develops ill feelings toward her brave husband. Oh desire, you are a destroyer, and you are poisonous. Leave me, just as the pregnant cow leaves the bull."[8]

You may address your prayers to the five elements, or any other object of your faith, with the following simple mantras:

OM SHANTI KĀMA
OM SHANTI KRODHA
OM SHANTI MOHA
OM SHANTI LOBHA

You should repeat each of these mantras several times. It is especially beneficial to repeat them when you feel overtaken by any of the four negative attributes, or if your actions are impelled by desire or anger.

You must realize that santoṣa (the sense of satisfaction and contentment) is the greatest of treasures you can have. If you have worldly possessions, basic comforts, and other possibilities of enjoyment, but do not have santoṣa, you will be unhappy in spite of everything. Make an effort to fight the four enemies. Do not let them damage you. Strive for a mental state of santoṣa, which will bring radiation to your face and make your mind and body strong.

HEALING WITH SEXUAL ENERGY

Sexual energy is usually channeled to experience momentary pleasure. This energy is very powerful as we discussed in the previous section. Sexual energy can also be channeled for healing. For doing so, you simply visualize the ailing or weak part at the moment of sexual pleasure. You have to make a channel between the concentrated energy, which you enjoy in the form of sensuous pleasure, and the ailing part of yourself. This can be done only by

---

[8] *Athārvaveda*, VII, 113.

concentrating your mind upon the ailing part at the moment you feel the concentration of sexual energy. It is not something that should be done in sequence, one after the other. The mind works very fast, and it is through your power of intellect that you are capable of directing the mind. In the present context, your thoughts are concentrated to the affected part instantly at the moment you experience sexual bliss. This is where you need to train your mind.

The concentration of energy that we call sexual bliss lasts for a very short time. We have discussed ways to prolong this bliss. You can train yourself to rapidly visualize the ailing part at the specific moment of bliss. This does not mean that you should think of the process of channeling the energy before you experience sexual bliss. If you do, you may make yourself tense, and may not be able to concentrate the energy for a sexual bliss. You can learn to trap this energy and direct it to the desired part during that brief moment when you reach the peak of the sexual activity. You cannot learn to do that in the absence of sexual energy. If you prepare yourself to trap this energy before it is there, you will lose yourself in the preparation and block the channels for the sexual energy. You should trap the energy just at that precise moment of the onset of the accumulation of sexual energy leading to bliss. Do not get lost in the sensuous pleasure and forget about the ailing part at that moment! If I talk too much of the technique, you will be preoccupied by the theory and will lose the mental concentration. Language is always insufficient to explain practices that are above the level of sensory perception. You will understand it as you try it and perfect the technique.

OM SHANTI

BIBLIOGRAPHY

Caraka Saṃhitā. An ancient Āyurvedic text. Translations in this book are by Prof. Priya Vrat Sharma.

Sheldrake, Rupert. *The Rebirth of Nature: The Greening of Science and God.* London: Century, 1990.

Spencer, Peter S., et al. "Lathyrism: Evidence for the Role of the Neuroexcitatory Aminoacid BOAA," in *Lancet.* Nov. 8, 1986.

The Vedas: Athārva, Sāma, R̥g, Yajur. References to these early Hindu works have been translated by the author.

Verma, Vinod. *Ayurveda: A Way of Life.* York Beach, ME: Samuel Weiser, 1995.

Verma, Vinod. *Yoga for Integral Health.* New Delhi: Hind Pocket Books, 1991.

Verma, Vinod. *Yoga Sūtras of Patañjali: A Scientific Exposition.* New Delhi: Clarion Books, 1993.

INDEX

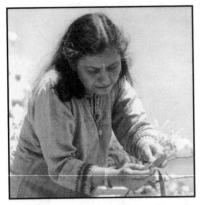

ABOUT THE AUTHOR

Dr. Vinod Verma was born into a family where yoga and Āyurveda were a part of everyday life. She learned yogic practices from her father, while Āyurveda was taught by her grandmother, who cured women and children. Despite this strong family tradition, Dr. Verma chose to study modern medical science and earned two doctorates: one in Reproduction Biology from Punjab University, and one in Neurobiology from Université de Pierre et Marie Curie, Paris. She pursued advanced research in neurobiology at the National Institutes of Health, Bethesda, MD, and continued her work at the Max-Planck Institut in Germany. At the peak of her career in medical research in a pharmaceutical company in Germany, Dr. Verma realized that the modern approach to healthcare is fragmented (non-holistic). In addition, Westerners are directing resources to cure diseases rather than maintaining health. In response, Dr. Verma founded NOW (The New Way Health Organization) to spread the message of holistic living, preventive methods for health care, and other self-help therapeutic measures.

Dr. Verma has been studying Āyurveda in the traditional style of *Guru-sisya* with Acharya Priya Vrat Sharma from the Benares Hindu University for the last twelve years. She is also researching the ethnic and folklore Āyurvedic tradition in order to bring the simple home remedies of Āyurveda to the West. In order to teach Āyurveda in the ancient tradition of the sages, Dr. Verma built a Himalayan center on the bank of the Ganges to include an Āyurvedic garden and a student home. She also has a center in New Delhi/Noida.

Dr. Verma has had numerous scientific papers published in international journals. Her five books on Āyurveda and yoga are published in various European languages. She has several other books in preparation. She lectures extensively, has appeared on German and Italian television to speak on the theme of holistic living and health, and is always happy to hear from readers.